Alexander Crever Abbott

The principles of bacteriology: a practical manual for students and

physicians

Alexander Crever Abbott

The principles of bacteriology: a practical manual for students and physicians

ISBN/EAN: 9783337214791

Printed in Europe, USA, Canada, Australia, Japan

Cover: Foto ©Paul-Georg Meister /pixelio.de

More available books at **www.hansebooks.com**

THE PRINCIPLES

OF

BACTERIOLOGY:

A PRACTICAL MANUAL FOR STUDENTS AND PHYSICIANS.

BY

A. C. ABBOTT, M.D.,

FIRST ASSISTANT, LABORATORY OF HYGIENE, UNIVERSITY OF PENNSYLVANIA, PHILADELPHIA.

WITH ILLUSTRATIONS.

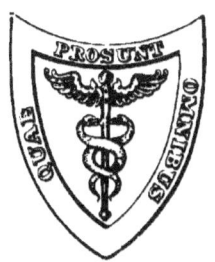

PHILADELPHIA:
LEA BROTHERS & CO.
1892.

Entered according to Act of Congress, in the year 1891, by
LEA BROTHERS & CO.,
In the Office of the Librarian of Congress at Washington, D. C.

PREFACE.

In preparing this book the author has kept in mind the needs of the student and practitioner of medicine, for whom the importance of an acquaintance with practical bacteriology cannot be overestimated.

It is to advances made through bacteriological research that we are indebted for much of our knowledge of the conditions underlying infection, and for the elucidation of many hitherto obscure problems concerning the etiology, the modes of transmission, and the means of prevention of infectious maladies.

Only within a comparatively short time have students and physicians been enabled to obtain the systematic instruction in this science that is of value in aiding them in their efforts to check disease. The rapid increase in the number who are availing themselves of these opportunities speaks directly for the practical value of the science.

As the majority of those undertaking the study of bacteriology do so with the view of utilizing it in medical practice, and as many of these can devote to it but a portion of their time, it is desirable that the subject-matter be presented in as direct a manner as possible.

Presuming the reader to be unfamiliar with the subject, the author has restricted himself to those fundamental features that are essential to its understanding. The object has been to present the important ideas and methods as concisely as is compatible with clearness, and at the same time to accentuate throughout the underlying principles which govern the work.

With the view of inducing independent thought on the part of the student, and of diminishing the frequency of that oft-heard query, "What shall I do next?" experiments have been suggested wherever it is possible. These have been arranged to illustrate the salient points of the work and to attract attention to the minute details, upon the observation of which so much in bacteriology depends.

A. C. A.

PHILADELPHIA, December, 1891.

CONTENTS.

INTRODUCTION.

"Omne vivum ex vivo"—The overthrow of the doctrine of spontaneous generation 13–21

CHAPTER I.

Definition of bacteria—Their place in nature—Difference between parasites and saprophytes—Nutrition of bacteria—Products of bacteria—Their relation to oxygen—Influence of temperature upon their growth . . . 22–28

CHAPTER II.

Morphology of bacteria—Grouping—Mode of multiplication—Spore-formation—Motility 29–36

CHAPTER III.

Principles of sterilization by heat—Different methods employed—Principles of discontinued sterilization—Sterilization under pressure—Apparatus employed . . 37–48

CHAPTER IV.

Disinfection—Antiseptics—Inorganic salts as disinfectants—The value of corrosive sublimate—Heat . . 49–53

CHAPTER V.

The principles involved in the methods of isolation of bacteria in pure culture by the plate method of Koch—Materials employed 54–58

CONTENTS.

CHAPTER VI.

Preparation of media—Bouillon, gelatin, agar-agar, potato, blood-serum, etc. 59–76

CHAPTER VII.

Preparation of the tubes, flasks, etc., in which the media are to be preserved 77–80

CHAPTER VIII.

Technique of making plates—Esmarch tubes, Petri plates, etc. 81–90

CHAPTER IX.

The incubator used in bacteriological work—Gas-pressure regulator—Thermo-regulator—The form of burner employed in heating the incubator 91–98

CHAPTER X.

The study of colonies—Their naked-eye peculiarities and their appearance under different conditions—Differences in the structure of colonies from different species of bacteria—Stab cultures–Slant cultures 99–103

CHAPTER XI.

Systematic study of an organism—Steps necessary in identifying an organism as a definite species . . . 104–121

CHAPTER XII.

Methods of staining—Solutions employed—Preparation and staining of cover-slips—Preparation of tissues for section-cutting—Staining of tissues—Special staining methods 122–150

CHAPTER XIII.

Inoculation of animals—Subcutaneous inoculation—Intra-venous injection 151–158

CHAPTER XIV.

Post-mortem examination of animals—Bacteriological examination of the tissues—Disposal of tissues and disinfection of instruments after the examination . . 159–163

CHAPTER XV.

Scheme for the complete study of an organism . . 164, 165

PRACTICAL APPLICATION OF THE METHODS OF BACTERIOLOGY.

CHAPTER XVI.

To obtain material upon which to begin work . . 167–170

CHAPTER XVII.

Various experiments in sterilization—Steam and hot-air methods of sterilizing 171–175

CHAPTER XVIII.

Bacteriological study of water, air, and soil—Methods of counting the colonies on the plates—Wolffhügel's counting apparatus—Sedgwick's method 176–191

CHAPTER XIX.

Inoculation experiments with sputum—Sputum septicæmia—Septicæmia resulting from the presence of the micrococcus tetragenus in the tissues—Tuberculosis . . 192–200

CHAPTER XX.

Tuberculosis—Microscopic appearance of miliary tubercles—Diffuse caseation—Cavity-formation—Encapsulation of tuberculous foci—Primary infection—Modes of infection—Location of the bacilli in the tissues—Staining peculiarities 201–216

CHAPTER XXI.

Suppuration—The staphylococcus pyogenes aureus . 217–224

CHAPTER XXII.

Typhoid fever—Study of the organism concerned in its production 225–231

CHAPTER XXIII.

Study of the bacillus of anthrax, and the effects produced by its inoculation into animals—Peculiarities of the organism under varying conditions of surroundings . 232–242

CHAPTER XXIV.

Bacteriology of diphtheria—Behavior of the bacillus diphtheriæ in the tissues of susceptible animals . . 243–252

CHAPTER XXV.

Experiments illustrating precautions to be taken in the study of disinfectants and antiseptics—Skin-disinfection . 253–257

BACTERIOLOGY.

INTRODUCTION.

"Omne vivum ex vivo"—The overthrow of the doctrine of spontaneous generation.

THE study of Bacteriology may be said to have had its birth with the observations made by Antony van Leeuwenhoek in the year 1675. Though it is during the past decade and a half that this line of research has received its greatest impulse, yet by a review of the developmental stages through which it has passed in its life of more than two centuries, we see that it has a most interesting and instructive history. From the very beginning its history is inseparably connected with the history of medicine, and as it now stands its relations to hygiene and preventive medicine are of the most important nature. It is, indeed, to a more intimate acquaintance with the biological activities of the micro-organisms that modern hygiene owes much of its value, and our knowledge upon infectious diseases has been developed to the position it now occupies. Though the contributions which have done most to place bacteriology on the footing of a science are those of recent years, still, during the earlier stages of its development, many observations were made which formed the foundation work for much that was to follow. Before regularly beginning our studies, therefore, it may be of advantage to acquaint ourselves with the more prominent of these investigations.

Antony van Leeuwenhoek, the first to describe the bodies now recognized as bacteria, was born at Delft, in Holland, in 1632. He was not considered a man of liberal education, having been during his early years an apprentice to a linendraper. During his apprenticeship he learned the art of lens-grinding, in which he became so proficient that he eventually perfected a lens by means of which he was enabled to see objects of much smaller dimensions than any hitherto seen with the microscopes in existence at that date. At the time of his discoveries he was following the trade of linendraper in Amsterdam.

In 1675 he published the fact that he had succeeded in perfecting a lens by means of which he could detect in a drop of rain water living, motile animalcules of the most minute dimensions—smaller than anything that had hitherto been seen. Encouraged by this discovery, he continued to examine various substances for the presence of what he considered animal life in its most minute form. He found in sea-water, in well-water, in the intestinal canal of frogs and birds, and in his own diarrhœal evacuations, objects that differentiated themselves the one from the other, not only by their shape and size, but also by the peculiarity of movement which some of them were seen to possess. In the year 1683 he discovered in the tartar scraped from between the teeth a form of microörganism upon which he laid special stress. This observation he embodied in the form of a contribution which was presented to the Royal Society of London on September 14, 1683. This paper is of particular importance, not only because of the careful, objective nature of the description given for the bodies seen by him, but also for the illustrations which accompany it. From a perusal of the text and an inspection of the plates there remains little room for doubt that Leeuwenhoek with his primitive lens had seen the bodies now recognized as bacteria.

Upon seeing these bodies he was apparently very much astonished, for he writes: "With the greatest astonishment I saw that everywhere through the material which I was examining were distributed animalcules of the most microscopic dimensions, which moved themselves about in a remarkably energetic way."

This observation was shortly followed by others of an equally important nature. His field of observation appears to have increased rapidly, for after a time he speaks of bodies of much smaller dimensions than those at first described by him.

Throughout all of Leeuwenhoek's work there is a conspicuous absence of the speculative. His contributions are marked by their purely objective nature.

After the presence of these organisms in water, in the mouth, and in the intestinal evacuations was made known to the world, it is hardly surprising that they were immediately seized upon as the explanation for the origin of many obscure diseases. So universal was the belief in a causal relation between these "animalcules" and disease, that it amounted almost to a germ mania. It became the fashion to suspect the presence of these organisms in all forms and kinds of disease, simply because they had been demonstrated in water.

Though nothing of value at the time had been done in the way of classification, and still less in separating and identifying the members of this large group, still, the foremost men of the day did not hesitate to ascribe to them not only the property of producing disease conditions, but some even went so far as to hold that variations in the appearance of the symptoms of disease were the result of differences in the behavior of the organisms in the tissues.

Marcus Antonius Plenciz, a physician of Vienna in 1762, expressed himself a firm believer in the work of Leeuwenhoek, and based the doctrine which he taught upon the discoveries of the Dutch observer, and upon observations of a confirmatory nature which he himself had made. The doctrine of Plenciz assumed a causal relation between the microörganisms discovered and described by Leeuwenhoek and all infectious diseases. He claimed that infection could be nothing else than a living substance, and endeavored on these grounds to explain the variations in the period of incubation for the different infectious diseases. He likewise believed the living contagium to be capable of multiplication within the body, and spoke of the possibility of its transmission through the air. He claimed a special germ for each disease, holding that just as from a given cereal only one kind of grain can grow, so by the special germ for each disease only that disease can be produced.

He found in all decomposing matters innumerable minute "animalculæ," and was so firmly convinced of their etiological relation to the process that he formulated the law: that decomposition can only take place when the decomposable material becomes coated with a layer of the organisms, and can proceed only when they increase and multiply.

However convincing the arguments of Plenciz appear,

they seem to have been lost sight of in the course of subsequent events, and by a few were even held in the light of productions from an unbalanced mind. For example, as late as 1820 we find Ozanam expressing himself on the subject as follows: " Many authors have written concerning the animal nature of the contagion of infectious diseases; many have indeed assumed it to be developed from animal substances and that it is itself animal, and possesses the property of life. I shall not waste time in efforts to refute these absurb hypotheses."

Similar expressions of opinion were heard from many other medical men of the time, all tending in the same direction, all doubting the possibility of these microscopic creatures belonging to the world of living things.

It was not until between the fourth and fifth decade of the present century that by the fortunate coincidence of a number of important discoveries the true relation of the lower organisms to infectious diseases was scientifically pointed out. With the investigations of Pasteur upon the cause of putrefaction in beer and the souring of wine; with the discovery by Pollender and Davaine of the presence of rod-shaped organisms in the blood of all animals dead of splenic fever, and the progress of knowledge upon the parasitic nature of certain diseases of plants, the old question of " contagium animatum" again began to receive attention. It was taken up by Henle, and it was he who first logically taught this doctrine of infection.

The main point, however, which had occupied the attention of scientific men from time to time for a period of about two hundred years subsequent to Leeuwenhoek's discoveries, was the origin of these bodies. Do they generate spontaneously, or are they the descendants of preëxisting creatures of the same kind? was the all-important question. Among the participants in this discussion were many of the most prominent men of the day.

In 1749 Needham, who held firmly to the opinion that the bodies which were creating such a general interest developed spontaneously, as the result of vegetative changes in the substances in which they were found, attempted to demonstrate by experiment the grounds upon which he held this view. He maintained that the bacteria which were seen to appear around a grain of barley which was allowed to germinate in a watch-crystal of water, which had been carefully covered, were the result of changes in the barley-grain itself, incidental to its germination.

Spallanzani, in 1769, drew attention to the laxity of the methods employed by Needham, and demonstrated that if infusions of decomposable vegetable matter were placed in flasks, which were then hermetically sealed, and the flasks and their contents allowed to remain for some time in a vessel of boiling water, neither living organisms could be detected nor would decomposition appear in the infusions so treated. The objection raised by Treviranus that the high temperature to which the infusions had been subjected had so altered them and the air about them, that the conditions favorable to spontaneous generation no longer existed, was met by Spallanzani by gently tapping one of the flasks that had been boiled, against some hard object until a minute crack was produced; invariably organisms and decomposition appeared in the flask thus treated.

From the time of the experiments of Spallanzani until as late as 1836 but little advance was made in the elucidation of this obscure problem.

In 1836 Schulz attracted attention to the subject by the convincing nature of his investigations. He showed that if the air which gained access to boiled infusions was robbed of its living organisms by being caused to pass through strong acid or alkaline solutions, no decomposition appeared and living organisms could not be detected in the infusions. Following quickly upon this contribution came Schwann, in 1837, and somewhat later (1854) Schröder and Dusch, with similar results obtained by somewhat different means. Schwann deprived the air which passed to his infusions of its living particles by passing it through highly-heated tubes; whereas Schröder and Dusch, by means of cotton-wool interposed between the boiled infusion and the outside air, robbed the air passing to the infusions of its organisms by the simple process of filtration. In 1860 Hoffmann and in 1861 Chevreul and Pasteur demonstrated that the precautions taken by the preceding investigators for rendering the air which entered these flasks free from bacteria were not necessary; that all that was necessary to prevent the access of bacteria to the infusions in the flasks was to draw out the neck of the flask into a fine tube, bend it down along the side of the flask and then bend it up again a few inches from its extremity, and leave the mouth open. The infusion was then to be boiled in the flask thus prepared and the mouth of the tube left open. The organisms which now fall into the tube will be arrested by the drop of water of condensation which collects at its lowest angle, and none can enter the flask.

Convincing though this work may seem, there still existed a number of doubters who required further proof that "spontaneous generation" was not the explanation for the mysterious appearance of these minute living objects, and it was not until some time later that Tyndall, in his well-known investigations upon the floating matters in the air, demonstrated again that the presence of living organisms in decomposing fluids was always to be explained either by the preëxistence of similar living forms in the infusion or upon the walls of the vessel containing it, or by the infusion having been exposed to air which had not been deprived of its organisms.

Throughout all the work bearing upon this subject, from the time of Spallanzani to that of Tyndall, certain irregularities were constantly appearing. It was found that certain substances required to be heated for a much longer time than was necessary to render other substances free from living organisms, and even under the most careful precautions decomposition would occasionally appear.

In 1762 Bonnet, who was deeply interested in this subject, had suggested, in reference to the results obtained by Needham, the possibility of the existence of "germs, or their eggs," which have the power to resist the temperature to which some of the infusions employed in Needham's experiments had been subjected.

More than a hundred years after Bonnet had made this purely speculative suggestion, it became the task of Ferdinand Cohn, of Breslau, to demonstrate its accuracy.

Cohn repeated the foregoing experiments with like results. He concluded that the irregularities could only be due to, either the existence of more resistant species of bacteria or to more resistant stages into which certain bacteria have the property of passing. After much work he demonstrated that certain of the rod-shaped organisms possess the power of passing into a resting or spore stage in the course of their life history, and when in this stage they are much less susceptible to the deleterious action of high temperatures than when they are growing as normal vegetative forms. With the discovery of these more resistant spores, the doctrine of spontaneous generation received its final blow. It was no longer difficult to explain the irregularities in the foregoing experiments, or was it any longer to be doubted that putrefaction and fermentation were the result of bacterial life and not the cause of it, and that these bacteria were the offspring from preëxisting similar forms. In other words, the law of Harvey, *Omne vivum ex ovo*, or its modification, *Omne vivum ex vivo*, was shown to apply, not only to the more highly organized members of the animal and vegetable kingdoms, but to the most microscopic, unicellular creatures as well.

Note.—I have presented only the most prominent investigations which aided in overthrowing the doctrine of spontaneous generation. For a more detailed account of this work the reader is referred to Löffler's *Vorlesungen über die geschichtliche Entwickelung der Lehre von den Bacterien*, upon which I have drawn largely in preparing the foregoing sketch.

CHAPTER I.

Definition of bacteria—Their place in nature—Difference between parasites and saprophytes—Nutrition of bacteria—Products of bacteria—Their relation to oxygen—Influence of temperature upon their growth.

By the term bacteria is understood that large group of minute vegetable organisms which multiply by a process of transverse division. They are spherical, oval, rod-like, and spiral in shape, and are commonly devoid of chlorophyll.[1] Owing to the absence of chlorophyll from their composition the bacteria are forced to either a saprophytic[2] or parasitic[3] form of existence.

Their life processes are so rapid and energetic that they result in the most profound alterations in the structure and composition of the materials upon which they are developing.

Decomposition and fermentation result from the presence of the saprophytic bacteria, while the changes

---

[1] Chlorophyll is the green coloring matter possessed by the higher plants by means of which they are enabled in the presence of sunlight to decompose carbonic acid (CO_2) and ammonia (NH_3) into their elementary constituents.

[2] A saprophyte is an organism that obtains its nutrition from dead organic matter.

[3] A parasite lives always at the expense of some other living, organic creature, and in the strictest sense of the word cannot exist upon dead matter. There exist, however, a group of so-called "facultative" saprophytes and parasites which possess the power of accommodating themselves to existing surroundings—at one time leading a parasitic, at another time a saprophytic form of existence.

brought about in the tissues of their host by the pure parasitic forms, find expression in disease processes and not unfrequently complete death.

The rôle played in nature by the saprophytic bacteria is a very important one. Through their presence the highly complicated tissues of dead animals and vegetables are resolved into the simpler compounds, carbonic acid and ammonia, in which form they may be taken up and appropriated as nutrition by the more highly organized members of the vegetable kingdom. It is to this ultimate production of carbonic acid, ammonia, and water by the bacteria, as end-products in the processes of decomposition and fermentation of the dead animal and vegetable tissues, that the demands of growing vegetation for these compounds can be supplied.

The chlorophyll plants do not possess the power of obtaining their carbon and nitrogen from such highly organized and complicated substances as serve for the nutrition of the bacteria, and as the production of these simpler compounds (CO_2, NH_3, H_2O) by the animal world is not sufficient to meet the demands of the chlorophyll plants, the importance of the part played by the bacteria in making up this deficit cannot be overestimated. Were it not for the activity of these microscopic living particles, all life upon the surface of the earth would certainly cease. Deprive higher vegetation of the carbon and nitrogen supplied to it as a result of bacterial activity, and its development comes rapidly to an end. Rob the animal kingdom of the food-stuffs supplied to it by the vegetable world, and life is no longer possible.

It is plain, therefore, that the saprophytes, which represent by far the large majority of all bacteria, must be looked upon by us in the light of benefactors, without which existence would be impossible.

With the parasites, on the other hand, the conditions are far from analogous. Through their existence there is constantly a loss, rather than a gain, to both the animal and vegetable kingdoms. Their host must always be a living body in which exist conditions favorable to their development and from which they appropriate substances which are necessary to the health and life of the tissues of the organism to which they may have found access. At the same time the substances which they form as products of their nutrition are direct poisons for the surrounding tissues.

In their relations to humanity the positions occupied by the two biologically different groups, the saprophytes on the one hand and the parasites on the other, are diametrically opposite. The saprophytic forms standing in the relation of benefactors, in resolving dead animal and vegetable bodies into their component parts, which serve for food for living vegetation, and, at the same time, removing from the surface of the earth the remains of all dead organic substances; while the parasitic group exist only at the expense of the more highly organized members of both kingdoms. It is to the parasitic group that the pathogenic[1] organisms belong.

In addition to the saprophytes which are concerned in the changes to which allusion has just been made, there exist other saprophytic forms which are recognized by their property of producing pigments of different color. These are known as the chromogenic[2] forms.

---

[1] Pathogenic organisms are those which possess the property of producing disease.

[2] Chromogenic, possessing the property of producing color.

NUTRITION OF BACTERIA.

Just what their exact rôle in nature is, it is difficult to say; but it is probable that in addition to their most conspicuous function of color production, they are also in some way concerned in the great process of disintegration which is constantly going on in all dead organic substances.

We know that through the agency of chlorophyll, in the presence of sunlight, the green plants are enabled to obtain the amount of nitrogen and carbon which is necessary to their growth from such simple bodies as carbon dioxide and ammonia, which they decompose into their elementary constituents. The bacteria, on the other hand, owing to the absence of chlorophyll from their tissues, do not possess this power. They must have their carbon and nitrogen presented as such, in the form of decomposable organic compounds.

In general, the bacteria obtain their nitrogen most readily from soluble albumins, and, to a certain degree, but by no means so easily, from salts of ammonia. In some of Nägeli's experiments it appeared probable that they could obtain the necessary amount of nitrogen from the salts of nitric acid. At all events, he was able in certain cases to demonstrate a reduction of nitric to nitrous acid, and ultimately to ammonia. Nevertheless, in all of these experiments circumstances point to the probability that the nitrogen obtained by the bacteria for building up their tissues in the course of their development, was derived from some source other than that of the nitric acid or the nitrites, and that the reduction of this acid was most probably a secondary phenomenon.

For the supply of carbon, many of the carbon compounds serve as sources upon which the bacteria can draw. The carbon deficit, for example, can be obtained from sugar and bodies of like composition; from glycerine and many of the fatty acids; and from the alkaline salts of tartaric, citric, malic, lactic, and acetic acids. In some instances carbon compounds which when present in concentrated form inhibit the growth of the lower organisms, may, when highly diluted, serve as nutrition for these bodies. Salicylic acid and ethyl alcohol come under this head.

In addition to carbon and nitrogen, water is essential to the life and development of bacteria. Without it no development occurs, and in many cases drying the organisms results in their death. Certain forms, on the contrary, though incapable of multiplying when in the dry stage, may be completely deprived of their water without causing them to lose the power of reproduction when favorable conditions present.

The closer study of the bacteria, and a more intimate acquaintance with their nutritive changes, demonstrate an appreciable variability in the character of the substances best suited for the nutrition of different species, one requiring a more concentrated form of nutrition, while another needs but a very limited amount of proteid substance for its development. Certain members bring about most profound alterations in the media in which they exist, while others produce but little apparent change. In one case alterations in the reaction of the media will be most conspicuous, while in another no such variation can be detected. With certain forms oxygen is essential for the proper performance of their functions, while with another group no evidence of life can be detected under the access of oxygen, and in a third group oxygen appears to play but an unimportant part, for development occurs as well with as without it. In the case of certain of the chromogenic forms the presence or absence of oxygen has a very decided effect upon the production of the pigments by which they are characterized.

For the normal development of bacteria it is not only essential that the sources from which they can obtain the necessary nutritive elements should exist, but account must also be taken of the products of growth of the organism in these substances. Nitrogen and carbon compounds in the proper form to be taken up and appropriated by the organism may exist in sufficient quantities, and still the growth of the organism after a very short time be entirely checked, owing to the production during their growth of substances inhibitory to their further development. Most conspicuous are the changes produced by the growing bacteria in the reaction of the media. Since the majority of these bodies grow best in media of a neutral or very slightly alkaline reaction, any excessive production of alkalinity or acidity, as a product of growth, arrests development, and no evidence of life or further multiplication can be detected until this deviation from the neutral reaction has been corrected.

Most favorable for the development of bacteria are neutral or very slightly alkaline solutions of albumin in one form or another.

Of considerable importance and interest in the study of the nutritive changes of bacteria is the difference in their relation to oxygen. It was Pasteur who first demonstrated the existence of species in the bacteria family which not only grow and multiply and perform definite physiological functions without the aid of oxygen, but to the existence of which oxygen is positively harmful. To these he gave the name of "anaërobic" bacteria in contradistinction to another group for the proper performance of whose functions oxygen is essential, which he called "aërobic" bacteria. In addition to these, there is a third group for the maintenance of whose existence the absence or presence of oxygen is apparently of no moment—their development progresses as well with as without it; these represent the class known as "facultative" in their relation to this gas. It is in this third group, the facultative, that the majority of bacteria belong. Though the multiplication of the facultative varieties is not interfered with by either the presence or absence of oxygen, yet experiments show that the products of their growth are different under the varying conditions of absence or presence of this gas.

Another element which plays a most important part in the biological functions of these organisms is the temperature under which they exist. The extremes of temperature under which bacteria are known to grow range from 5.5° C. to 48° C. At the former temperature development is hardly appreciable, it becomes more and more active until 38° C. is reached, when it is at its optimum, and, as a rule, ceases with 43° C. Neither of the extremes can be considered normal temperatures for the growth of these organisms. The most favorable temperature for the development of the majority of bacteria is that of the human body, viz., 37.5° C.

In general it may be said that for the growth and development of bacteria, organic matter of a neutral or slightly alkaline reaction, in the presence of moisture and at a suitable temperature, is necessary. From this can be formed some idea of the omnipresence in nature of these minute vegetable forms. Everywhere that these conditions exist, bacteria can be found.

CHAPTER II.

Morphology[1] of the bacteria—Grouping—Mode of multiplication—Spore-formation—Motility.

IN form the bacteria are unicellular, and are seen to exist as spherical, rod- or spindle-shaped bodies. They always develop from preëxisting cells of the same character and never appear spontaneously.

The classifications of the older authors were upon purely morphological peculiarities, and in consequence, were more or less complicated. The present tendency is to simplify this morphological classification, and to bring the bacteria into three great groups, with their subdivisions; each group comprising those members whose individual outline is that either of a sphere, a rod, or a spiral.

To these three grand divisions are given the names cocci or micrococci, bacilli, and spirilli.

In the group *micrococci* belong all spherical forms, *i. e.*, all those forms the individual members of which are of equal diameter in all directions.

The *bacilli* comprise all oval or rod-formed bacteria.

To the *spirilli* belong all organisms which are twisted in the form of a corkscrew.

The micrococci are subdivided according to their grouping, as seen in growing cultures: into *staphylococci*—those growing in masses like fish-roe or clusters of grapes; *streptococci*—those growing in chains con-

[1] Morphology, pertaining to shape; outline.

sisting of a number of individual cells strung together like beads or pearls upon a string; *diplococci*—those growing in pairs; *tetrads*—those developing as fours, and *sarcinæ*—those dividing into fours, eights, etc., as cubes—that is, in contra-distinction to all other forms, the segmentation, which is rarely complete, takes place in three directions of space, so that when growing, the bundle of segmenting cells presents somewhat the appearance of a bale of cotton.

To the bacilli belong all rod-shaped organisms, *i. e.*, those in which one diameter is always greater than the other.

In this group are found those organisms the life cycle of many of which present deviations from the simple rod shape. Many of them in the course of development increase in length into long threads along the course of which traces of segmentation may usually be found— the anthrax bacillus and bacillus subtilis are conspicuous examples of this. Again others, under certain conditions, possess the property of forming within the body of the rods oval, glistening spores, and if the conditions are not altered the rods may entirely disappear, so that nothing may be left in the culture but these oval forms. Again, many of them, from unfavorable conditions of nutrition, aëration, or temperature undergo pathological changes—that is, the individuals themselves experience alterations in their protoplasm which result in distortion of their outline. This is the production of the so-called "involution forms." But in all of these conditions, so long as death has not actually occurred, it is possible under favorable conditions to cause these forms to revert to the original rod-shaped bacilli from which they originated.

It must be borne in mind, however, that it is never possible by any means to bring about changes in these organisms that will result in the permanent conversion of the morphology of the members of one group into that of another—that is, one can never produce bacilli from micrococci or *vice versa*, and any evidence which may be presented to the contrary is based upon inaccurate methods of work.

Not infrequently bacilli may be observed irregularly massed together as a pellicle. When in this condition they are held together by a gelatinous material, and are known as zoöglœa of bacilli.

Very short oval bacilli may sometimes be mistaken for micrococci, and at times micrococci in the stage of segmentation into diplococci may be mistaken for short bacilli; but by careful inspection it will always be possible to detect a continuous outline along the sides of the former and a slight transverse indentation or partition-formation between the segments of the latter. The high index of refraction of spores, the property which gives to them their glistening appearance, will always serve to distinguish them from micrococci. This difference in refraction will be especially noticed if the illumination from the reflector of the microscope with which they are to be examined is reduced to the smallest possible bundle of light-rays. The spores, moreover, take up the staining reagents much less readily than do the micrococci. The crucial test, however, is the property, in the case of the spores, of growing out into bacilli; and of the spherical organism with which it has been confounded, of developing only into another micrococcus of the same round form.

For convenience, a common classification of the bacilli

is that based upon constant characteristics which are seen to appear in the course of their development under special conditions—certain of them possessing the power of forming spores, while from others this peculiarity is absent.

As yet but little is known of the life history of the spiral forms. Efforts toward their cultivation under artificial conditions have thus far been unsuccessful. Morphologically, they are thread- or rod-like bodies which are twisted into the form of spirals. In some of them the turns of the spiral are long, in others quite short. They are motile, and multiply apparently by the simple process of fission.[1]

The micrococci develop by simple fission. When development is in progress a single cell will be seen to elongate slightly in one of its diameters. Over the center of the long axis thus formed will appear a slight indentation in the outer envelope of the cell; this indentation will increase in extent until there exist eventually two individuals which are distinctly spherical, as was the parent from which they sprang, or they will remain together for a time as diplococci. The surfaces now in juxtaposition are flattened against one another, and not infrequently a fine, pale dividing line may be seen between the two cells. A similar division in the other direction will now result in the formation of a group of forms as tetrads. This, in short, is the method of multiplication of the micrococci.

In the formation of the staphylococci such division occurs irregularly in all directions, resulting in the production of the clusters in which these organs are com-

---

[1] Dividing into two transversely.

monly seen. With the streptococci, however, the tendency is for the segmentation to continue in one direction only, resulting in the production of the long chains of 4, 8, and 12 individuals.

The sarcinæ divide more or less regularly in three directions of space, but instead of becoming separated the one from the other as single cells, the tendency is for the segmentation to be incomplete. The cells remain together in masses and the indentations upon these masses or cubes which indicate the point of incomplete fission give to these bundles of cells the appearance commonly ascribed to them—that of a bale of cotton or packet of rags.

The multiplication of the bacilli is in the main similar to that given for the micrococci. A dividing cell will elongate slightly in the direction of its long axis; an indentation will appear about midway between its poles, and will become deeper and deeper until eventually two daughter cells will be formed. This process may occur in such a way that the two young bacilli will adhere together by their adjacent ends in much the same way that sausages are seen to be held together in strings, or the segmentation may take place more at right angles to the long axis, so that the proximal ends of the young cells are flattened while the distal extremities may be rounded or slightly pointed. In the anthrax bacillus, with which we are subsequently to become more intimately acquainted, the segmentation, when completed, results in an indentation of the adjacent extremities of the young segments, so that by the aid of high magnifying powers these surfaces are seen to be actually concave in their outline. Bacilli never divide longitudinally.

With the spore-forming bacilli, under favorable conditions of nutrition and temperature, the same process is seen to occur, but so soon as these conditions become altered, either by the exhaustion of the nutrition, the presence of detrimental substances, unfavorable temperatures, etc., there appears the stage in their life cycle to which we have referred as "spore-formation." This is the process by which the organisms are enabled to enter a stage in which they resist deleterious influences to a much higher degree than is possible for them when in the growing or vegetative condition.

In the spore, resting, or permanent stage, as it is called, no evidence of life whatever is given by the spores, though as soon as the conditions which favor their germination have been renewed, these spores develop again into the same kind of cells as those from which they originated, and the appearances observed in the vegetative or growing stage of their history are again to be seen.

Multiplication of spores, as such, does not occur. They possess the power of developing into individual rods of the same nature as those from which they were formed, but not of giving rise to a direct reproduction of spores.

When the conditions which favor spore-formation present, the protoplasm of the vegetative cells is seen to undergo a change. It loses its normal homogeneous appearance and becomes marked here and there by granular, refractive points of irregular shape and size. These eventually coalesce and leave the remainder of the cell clear and transparent. When this coalescence of highly refractive particles is complete the spore is perfected. In appearance, the spore is oval or round, very highly refractive, and of a glistening appearance. It is easily differentiated from the remainder of the cell, which now consists only of a cell-membrane and a perfectly transparent, clear fluid which surrounds the spore. Eventually both the cell-membrane and its fluid contents disappear, leaving the oval spore free in the medium in which it has been formed.

The spore, when perfectly developed, is highly glistening, oval in contour, and has the appearance of being surrounded by a dark, sharply defined border. It possesses no motion other than the mechanical tremor common to all insoluble microscopic particles suspended in fluids, and it remains quiescent until conditions favorable to its subsequent development into the vegetative form from which it originated, appear. Occasionally the membrane of the vegetative cell in which the spore is formed does not disappear from around it, and the spore may then be seen lying in a very delicate tubular envelope. Now and then remnants of the envelope may be noticed adhering to the spore which has not yet become completely free.

When stained, the spore-containing cells do not take up the dyes in a homogeneous way. By the ordinary methods the spores do not stain, so that they appear in the stained cells as pale, transparent, oval bodies, surrounded by the remainder of the cell, which has taken up the staining.

A single cell produces but one spore. This may be located either at an extremity or in the centre of the cell.

Occasionally spore-formation is accompanied by an enlargement of the cell at the point at which the process is in progress. As a result, the outline of the cell loses its regular rod shape and becomes that of a club, a drum-stick, or a lozenge, depending upon whether the location of the spore is to be at the pole or in the centre of the cell.

In addition to the property of spore-formation there is another striking difference between the members of the rod-shaped organisms, namely, the property of motility which many of them are seen to possess. This power of motion is due to the possession by the motile bacilli of very delicate, hair-like appendages or flagellæ, by the lashing motions of which the rods possessing them are propelled through the fluid. In some cases the flagellæ come off from but one end of a bacillus, either singly or in a bunch; again, they may be seen at both poles, and in some cases, especially with the bacillus of typhoid fever, they are given off from the whole surface of the rod.

For a long time the motility of certain of the bacteria was supposed to be due to the possession of some such form of locomotive apparatus because similar appendages had been seen in certain of the large motile spirillæ found in stagnant water, but it was not until very recently that the accuracy of this suspicion was actually demonstrated. By a special method of staining, Löffler has been able, in a number of cases, to render visible these hair-like appendages. His method consists in the employment of a mordant, by the aid of which the flagellæ are caused to retain the staining, and thus become visible. Löffler's method of staining will be found in the chapter devoted to this part of the technique.

CHAPTER III.

Principles of sterilization by heat—Different methods employed—Principles of discontinued sterilization—Sterilization under pressure—Apparatus employed.

By the term sterilization, as employed here, is understood the destruction of bacteria by heat. It is accomplished in two ways: either by dry heat, or by moist heat in the form of steam.

Experiments have taught us that the process of sterilization by dry heat has a relatively limited application because of its many disadvantages. For successful sterilization by the method of dry heat, not only is a relatively high temperature essential, but the substances under treatment must be exposed to this temperature for a comparatively long time. Its penetrating action into the substances which are to be sterilized is, moreover, much less energetic than that of steam. Many substances of vegetable and animal origin are rendered useless by subjection to the dry method of sterilization. For these reasons there are comparatively few substances which may be sterilized in this way without serious damage to their further usefulness.

Successful sterilization by dry heat cannot usually be accomplished at a temperature lower than 150° C., and to this degree of heat must the objects be subjected for not less than one hour. For the sterilization, therefore, of the organic materials of which the media employed in bacteriological work are composed, and of domestic articles, such as cotton, woollen, wooden, and leather articles, this method is entirely impracticable. In bacteriological work its application is limited to the sterilization of glass-ware principally—such, for example, as flasks, plates, small dishes, test-tubes, pipettes—and such metal instruments as are not seriously injured by the high temperature.

With sterilization by moist heat—steam—the conditions are much more favorable. The penetrating action of the steam is not only much more energetic, but the temperature at which this is ordinarily accomplished is, as a rule, not destructive in its action. This is conspicuously seen in the work of the laboratory. The culture media, composed in the main of decomposable organic materials, which would be rendered entirely worthless if exposed to the dry method of sterilization, sustain no injury whatever when intelligently subjected to an equally effective sterilization with steam. The same may be said of cotton and woollen fabrics, bedding, clothing, etc.

Aside from the relations of the two methods to the materials to be sterilized, their action toward the organisms to be destroyed is quite different. The penetrating action of the steam renders it by far the more efficient agent of the two. The spores of several organisms which are killed by an exposure of but a few moments to the action of steam, resist the destructive action of dry heat at a higher temperature for a much greater length of time.

These differences will be strikingly brought out in the experimental work on this subject. For our purposes it is necessary to say that the two methods have the following applications:

The dry method, at a temperature of 150°–180° C., for one hour, is employed for the sterilization of glass-ware: flasks, test-tubes, culture dishes, pipettes, plates, etc.

The sterilization by steam is practised with all media, whether fluid or solid. Bouillon, milk, gelatin, agar-agar, potato, etc., are under no conditions to be subjected to the dry heat.

The methods by which heat is employed in processes of sterilization vary with circumstances. In its employment as dry heat its application is always continuous —*i. e.*, the objects to be sterilized are simply exposed to the proper temperature for the length of time necessary to destroy all living organisms which may be upon them. With steam, on the other hand, the objects to be sterilized are frequently of such a nature that a prolonged application of the heat would materially injure them. For this reason steam is usually applied intermittently and for short periods of time. The principles involved in this method of sterilization depend upon differences of resistance toward heat which the organisms to be destroyed are seen to possess at different stages of their development. During the life history of many of the bacilli there is a time in which the resistance of the organism toward the action of both chemical and thermal agents is much higher than at other stages of its development. This increased power of resistance is seen to exist when these organisms are in the *spore* or *resting stage*, to which reference has already been made. When in the vegetative or growing stage, most of these organism are killed in a short time by a relatively low temperature, whereas, when conditions have arisen which favor the production of spores, these spores are seen to be capable of resisting very much higher temperatures for an appreciably longer time. These differences in resistance toward heat which the spore-forming organisms are seen to possess at their different stages of development, are taken advantage of in the process of sterilization by steam which is known as the *fractional* or *intermittent method*, and form the principle on which the method is based.

The object aimed at in this method is to destroy the organisms in the shortest time and with the least amount of heat. It is accomplished by subjecting them to the elevated temperature at the time when they are in the vegetating or growing stage—*i. e.*, the stage at which they are least resistant. In order to accomplish this it is necessary that there should exist conditions of temperature, nutrition, and moisture which favor the vegetation of the bacilli, and the germination of any spores that may be present. When these surroundings are found, the spore-forming organisms are not only less likely to go into the spore stage than when their environments are less favorable to their vegetation, but spores which may already exist develop very quickly into mature cells.

It is plain, then, that with the first application of the steam to the substance to be sterilized, the mature vegetative forms of these organisms are destroyed, while certain spores which might have been present resist this treatment, providing the sterilization has not been continued for too long a time. If now the sterilization is discontinued, and the material which presents conditions favorable to the germination of the spores is allowed to stand for a time, usually for about twenty-four hours, at a temperature of from $30°-35°$ C., those spores which resisted the action of the steam will in the course of this time germinate into the less resistant vegetative cells,

A second short exposure to the steam kills these forms in turn, and by a repetition of this process all organisms which were present may be destroyed without the application of the steam having been at any time of long duration. In this process the usual plan is to subject the materials to be sterilized to the action of steam, under the normal conditions of temperature and pressure, for fifteen minutes on each of three successive days, and during the intervening days to retain them at a temperature of about 25°–30° C. At the end of this time all living organisms which were present will have been destroyed, and unless opportunity is given for the access of new organisms from without, the substances thus treated remain sterile.

It must be borne in mind that this method of sterilization is only applicable in those cases which present conditions favorable to the germination of the spores into mature vegetative cells. Dry substances or organic materials in which decomposition is far advanced, where the proper conditions for the germination of spores are not present, cannot be successfully sterilized by the intermittent method.

The process of fractional sterilization at *low* temperatures is based upon exactly the same principle, but differs in two respects, viz., it requires a longer time for its accomplishment, and the temperature at which it is conducted is not raised above 68°–70° C. It is employed for the sterilization of easily decomposable materials, which would be rendered useless by the temperature of steam, but which remain intact at the temperature employed. This process requires that the material to be sterilized should be subjected to a temperature of 68°–70° C. for one hour on each of six successive days, an interval of twenty-four hours being allowed between the exposures to this temperature for the germination of spores into mature cells. During this interval the substances under treatment are kept at about 25°–30° C. The temperature employed in this process suffices to destroy the vitality of almost all organisms in the vegetative stage in about one hour. Blood-serum is always sterilized by the intermittent method at low temperature.

Sterilization by steam is also practised by what may be called the direct method. That is to say, both the mature organisms and the spores which may be present in the material to be sterilized are destroyed by a single exposure to the steam. In this method steam at its ordinary temperature and pressure—live steam or streaming steam as it is called—is employed just as in the first method described, but it is allowed to act for a much longer time, usually not less than one hour. Or, steam under pressure, and consequently of a higher temperature, is now frequently employed. In this method a single exposure of fifteen minutes is sufficient for the destruction of all bacilli and their spores, providing the pressure of the steam is not less than one atmosphere over and above that of normal—this is equivalent to an approximate temperature of 122° C. to which the organisms are exposed.

The objection to both of these methods of direct sterilization by steam is that many substances which it is desirable to retain in as near their normal condition as possible are materially altered by this energetic form of treatment. Gelatin is not only rendered cloudy, but loses the power of gelatinzing. Many of the other media contain always a fine precipitate after this method; in fact, for most of the media which we employ, the discontinued method at the temperature of streaming steam gives the most satisfactory results.

For sterilization by steam the apparatus commonly employed has until recently been the cylindrical boiler recommended by Koch, a cut of which may be seen in Fig. 1.

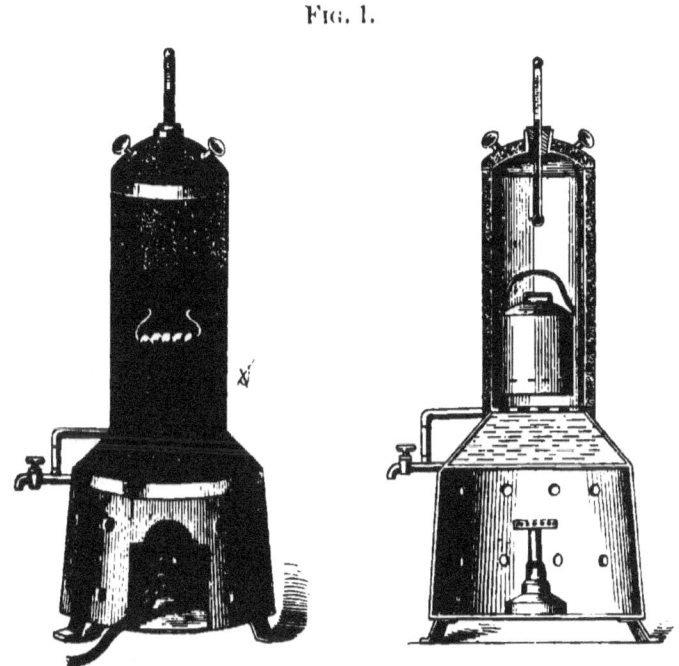

Fig. 1.

Its construction is very simple. It consists of a copper cylinder, the lower fourth of which is somewhat larger in diameter than the remaining three-fourths, and acts as a reservoir for the water from which the steam is to be generated. Covering this section of the cylinder is a wire rack or grating through which the steam passes, and which serves as a bottom upon which the materials to be sterilized rest. Above this, comprising the remaining three-fourths of the cylinder, is the chamber for the reception of the materials over and through which the steam is to pass. The cylinder is closed by a snugly-fitting cover through which are usually two perforations into which a thermometer and a manometer may be inserted. The whole of the outer surface of the apparatus is encased in a non-conducting mantle of asbestos or felt.

The water is heated by a gas-flame placed in an enclosed chamber, upon which the apparatus rests, which serves to diminish the loss of heat and deflection of the flame through the action of draughts. The apparatus is simple in construction, and the only point which is to be observed while using it is the level of the water in the reservoir. On the reservoir is a water-gauge which indicates at all times the amount of water in the apparatus. The amount of water should never be too small to be indicated by the gauge, otherwise there is danger of the reservoir becoming dry and the bottom of the apparatus being destroyed by the direct action of the flame.

A sterilizer now gaining favor for use in laboratories is an apparatus originally intended for use in the kitchen. It is the so-called "Arnold Steam Sterilizer." It is very ingenious in its construction as well as economical in its employment.

The difference between this apparatus and that just described is that it provides for the condensation of the steam after its escape from the sterilizing chamber, and returns the water of condensation automatically to the reservoir, so that in practice the apparatus requires but little attention, as with moderate care there is no fear of the water in the reservoir becoming exhausted and the consequent destruction of the sterilizer.

Fig. 2 gives an illustration of this apparatus.

FIG. 2.

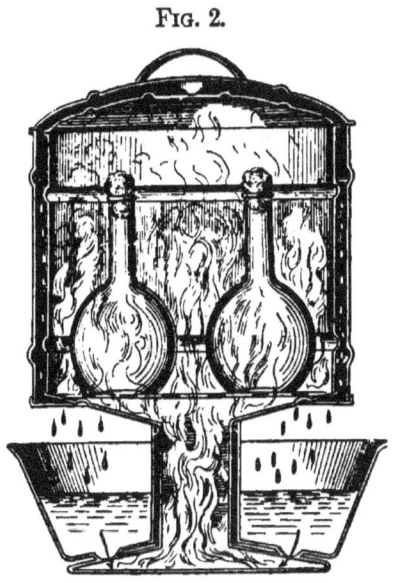

For sterilization by steam *under pressure* several special forms of apparatus exist. The principles of them all are, however, the same. They provide for the generation of steam in a chamber from which it cannot escape when the apparatus is closed. Upon the cover of this chamber is a safety-valve, which can be regulated so that any degree of pressure desirable can be maintained within the sterilizing chamber. These sterilizers are known as "digestors" and also by the French name "autoclav." Their construction can best be understood by reference to Fig. 3.

The dry sterilizers used in laboratories are simply double-walled boxes of Russian or Swedish iron (Fig. 4),

FIG. 3.

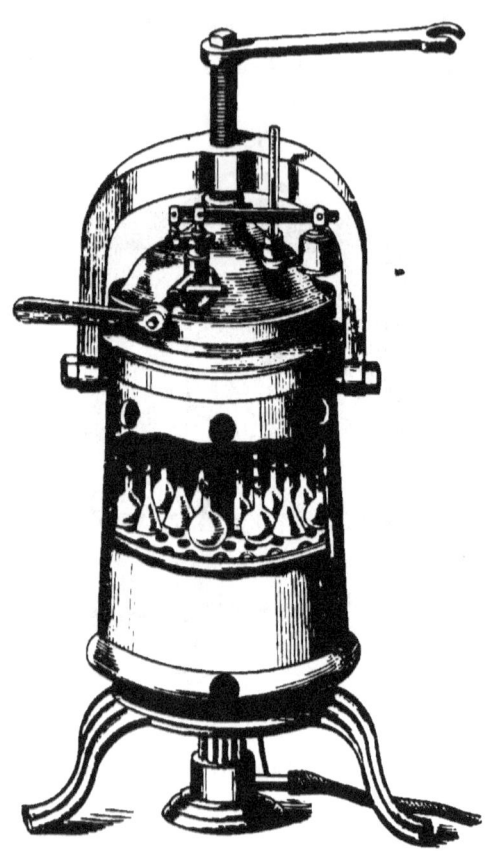

having a double-walled door, which closes tightly, and a heavy copper bottom. They are arranged with ventilating openings for the escape of the contained air and the entrance of the heated air. The flame, usually from a rose burner (Fig. 5), is applied directly to the bottom. The heat circulates from the lower surface around about the apparatus through the space between its walls.

The construction of the copper bottom of the apparatus upon which the flame impinges, is designed to prevent the direct action of the flame upon the sheet-iron bottom of the chamber. It consists of several copper plates placed one above the other, but with a space of about 4 to 5 mm. between the plates. These copper bottoms after a time become burned out, and unless they are replaced the apparatus is useless. The older form

Fig. 4.

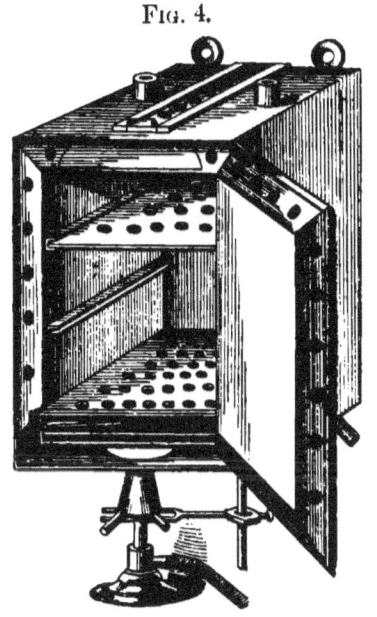

Fig. 5.

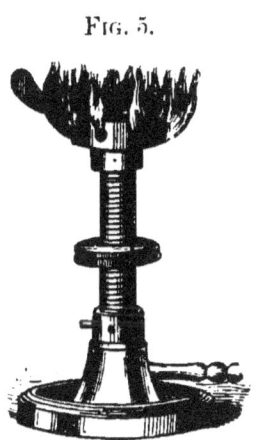

of sterilizers are so constructed that their repair is a matter involving some time and expense. To meet this objection I have had constructed a sterilizer in all respects similar to the old form except in the arrangement of this copper bottom. This is so made that it can be easily slipped in and out, so that by keeping several sets of copper plates on hand a new one can readily be slipped into the apparatus when the old one is burned out.

In the employment of the dry sterilizer care should

always be given to the condition of the copper bottom; for the direct application of the heat to the sheet-iron plate upon which the substances to be sterilized stand, results not only in destruction of the apparatus, but frequently in destruction of the substances undergoing sterilization.

Since the temperature at which this form of sterilization is usually accomplished is high—150° to 180° C.—it is well to have the apparatus encased in asbestos boards, to diminish the radiation of heat from its surfaces. This not only confines the heat to the apparatus, but guards against the destructive action of the radiated heat on woodwork, furniture, etc., that may be in the neighborhood.

CHAPTER IV.

Disinfection—Antiseptics—Inorganic salts as disinfectants—The value of corrosive sublimate—Heat.

IN contradistinction to sterilization, disinfection implies the destruction of bacteria by chemical processes. In the destruction of bacteria by means of chemical substances, there occurs most probably a definite chemical reaction ; that is to say, the characteristics of both the bacteria and the agent employed in their destruction are lost in the production of a third body, the result of their combination. It is impossible to say with absolute certainty, as yet, that this is the case, but the evidence that is rapidly accruing from the more recent studies upon disinfectants and their mode of action point strongly to the accuracy of this belief. This reaction, in which the typical structures of both bodies concerned is lost, takes place between the agent employed for disinfection and the protoplasm of the bacteria. For example, in the reaction that is seen to take place between the salts of mercury and albuminous bodies there results a third compound, which has neither the characteristics of mercury nor of albumin, but partakes of the peculiarities of both ; it is a combination of albumin and mercury known by the indefinite term "albuminate of mercury." Some such reaction as this occurs when the soluble salts of mercury are brought in contact with bacteria. This view has recently been strengthened by the experiments of Geppert, in which the reaction was caused to take place between the spores of the anthrax bacillus and a solution of mercuric chloride, the result being the apparent destruction of the living properties of the spores by the formation of this third compound. In these experiments it was shown that though this combination had taken place, still it did not of necessity imply the complete death of the protoplasm of the spores, for if by proper means the combination of mercury with their protoplasm was broken up, many of the spores returned from their condition of apparent death to that of life, with all their previous disease-producing and cultural peculiarities. Geppert employed a solution of ammonium sulphide for the purpose of destroying the combination of spore-protoplasm and mercury. The mercury was precipitated from the protoplasm as an insoluble sulphide, and the protoplasm of the spores returned to its original condition. These and other somewhat similar experiments have given an entirely new impulse to the study of disinfectants, and in the light shed by them many of our previously formed ideas concerning the action of disinfecting agents must be modified. The process is not a catalytic one—*i. e.*, occurring simply as a result of the presence of the disinfecting body which is not itself destroyed in its process of destruction—but is, as said, a definite chemical reaction which takes place within certain more or less fixed limits; that is to say, with a given amount of the disinfectant employed, just so much work, expressed in terms of disinfection—destruction of bacteria—can be accomplished.

Another point in favor of this view is the increased energy of the reaction with elevation of temperature. Just as in many other chemical phenomena, the intensity of the reaction becomes greater under the influence of heat, so in the process of disinfection the combination between the disinfectant and the organisms to be destroyed is much more energetic at a temperature of 37° to 39° C. than it is at 12° to 15° C.

What has been said refers more particularly to the inorganic salts which are employed for this purpose. It is probable that the organic bodies which possess disinfectant properties owe this power to some such similar reaction, though, as yet, these substances have not been so thoroughly studied in this relation.

The reaction between these inorganic salts and albuminous bodies is not a selective action; they combine in most instances with any or all protoplasmic bodies present. For this reason the efficacy of the practical application of many of the commonly employed disinfectants is a matter of grave doubt. For example, the disinfection of excreta, sputum, or blood containing pathogenic organisms, by means of corrosive sublimate, is a procedure of very questionable success. The amount of sublimate employed may be entirely used up and rendered inactive as a disinfectant by the ordinary protoplasmic substances present without having any appreciable effect upon the bacteria which may be in the mass.

These remarks are introduced in order to guard against the implicit confidence so often placed in the disinfecting value of corrosive sublimate. In bacteriological laboratories, where there is constantly more or less of infectious material, it is the custom, with few exceptions, to have vessels containing solutions of corrosive sublimate at hand, by which infectious materials may be rendered harmless. The value of this procedure, as we have just learned, is always more or less questionable, especially in those cases in which the substance to be disinfected is of an albuminous nature. With the introduction of such substances into the sublimate solution the mercury is quickly precipitated by the albumin and its disinfecting properties may be entirely destroyed; we may in a very short time have little else than water containing a precipitate of albumin and mercury, in so far as its value as a disinfectant is concerned.

In the laboratory, then, heat is the surest agent to employ. All tissues containing infectious organisms should be *burned*, and all cloths, test-tubes, flasks, and dishes should be boiled in 2 per cent. soda solution for fifteen to twenty minutes, or placed in the steam sterilizer for at least half an hour.

Intestinal evacuations may best be disinfected with *milk of lime*, a mixture composed of lime in solution and in suspension. This should be thoroughly mixed with the evacuations until the mass reacts distinctly alkaline, and should remain in contact with the infective substance for several hours.

Sputum in which tubercle bacilli are present, as well as the vessel containing it, must be boiled in soda solution for fifteen minutes or steamed in the sterilizer for at least half an hour.

On the whole, for the laboratory we should as yet rely more upon the destructive properties of heat than upon that of chemical agents.

From what has been said, the absurdity of sprinkling about, here and there, a little carbolic acid or in placing about apartments in which infectious diseases are in progress little vessels of carbolic acid, must be plain. The disinfection of water-closets and cesspools by allowing now and then a few cubic centimetres of some so-called disinfectant to trickle through the pipes is a failure. A disinfectant must be *applied to the bacteria, and must be in contact with them for a long enough time to insure the destruction of their life.* In the light of the latest experiments upon disinfectants, the place formerly occupied by many agents in the list of substances employed for the purpose will most likely be changed as they are studied more closely.

The agents, then, which will prove of most value in the laboratory for the purpose of rendering infectious materials harmless are: *Heat,* either by burning, by steaming for from half an hour to an hour, or by boiling in a 2 per cent. soda solution for fifteen minutes; a solution of *chlorinated lime* ("chloride of lime"), in which the percentage of chlorine is high; and *milk of lime.* The materials to be disinfected in either of the lime solutions should remain in them for several hours. The solutions should be freshly prepared when needed, as they rapidly decompose upon standing.

Antiseptic. An antiseptic is a body which, by its presence, prevents the growth of bacteria without of necessity killing them. A body may be an antiseptic without possessing disinfecting properties to any very high degree, but a disinfectant is always an antiseptic as well.

CHAPTER V.

The principles involved in the methods of isolation of bacteria in pure culture by the plate method of Koch—Materials employed.

SINCE the introduction of the plate method for isolating in pure culture the individual species from mixtures of bacteria, a number of modifications have been adopted, but the principle of them all is the same. The observation which led to their development was a very simple one, and one that is commonly before us. Koch noticed that on solid substances, such, for example, as a slice of potato, which had been exposed for a time to the air and which afforded proper nourishment for the lower organisms, there developed after a short time small patches of material which proved to be colonies of bacteria. Each of these colonies on closer examination showed itself to be, as a rule, composed of but a single species. There was no tendency toward a confluence of these colonies, and from the differences in their naked-eye appearances, it was easy to see that they were mostly the outgrowth of different species of bacteria.

The question that then presented itself was: If from a mixture of organisms floating in the air it is possible in this way to obtain in pure cultures the individual organisms composing the mixture, what means can be employed for obtaining the same results at will from mixtures of different organisms when found under other conditions?

It was plain that the organisms were to be distinguished, the one from the other, only by the structure and general appearance of the colonies growing from them, for upon their morphology alone this is impossible.

What means could be devised, then, for separating the individual members of a mixture, in such a way that they would remain in a fixed position, and be sufficiently widely separated, the one from the other, as not to interfere with the production of colonies of characteristic appearance, which would, under the proper conditions, develop from each individual cell?

If a test-tube of decomposed bouillon were poured out upon a large flat surface, the individual bacteria in the mass would be very much more widely separated the one from the other than they were when the bouillon was in the tube. But they are in a fluid medium, and there is no possibility of their either remaining separated or of their forming colonies under these conditions, so that it is impossible by this means to pick out the individuals in the mixture.

If, however, it is possible to find some substance which possesses the property of being at one time fluid and at another time solid, which can be added to this bouillon without in any way interfering with the life functions of the bacteria, then, as solidification sets in, the organisms will be fixed in their positions and the conditions will be analogous to that seen on the bit of potato.

Gelatin possesses this property. At a temperature which does not interfere with the life of the organisms it is quite fluid, whereas when subjected to a lower temperature it solidifies. When once solid it may be kept at a temperature favorable to the growth of the bacteria and retain its solid condition.

Gelatin was added to the fluids containing mixtures of bacteria, and the whole was then poured upon a large flat surface, allowed to solidify, and the results noted. It was found that the conditions seen on the slice of potato could be reproduced, that the individuals in the mixture of bacteria grew well in the gelatin, and, as on the potato, grew in colonies of typical macroscopic structure, so that they could easily be separated the one from the other by their naked-eye appearances. It was necessary, however, to use a more dilute mixture of bacteria than that seen in the original decomposed bouillon. The number of individuals in the tube was so enormous that on the gelatin plate they were so closely packed together that it was not only impossible to pick them out because of their proximity the one to the other, but also because this close packing together materially interfered with the production of those characters by means of which differences can be seen with the naked eye. The numbers of organisms were then diminished by a process of dilution, consisting of transferring a small portion of the original mixture into a second tube of sterilized bouillon to which gelatin had been added and liquefied; from this a similar portion was added to a third galatin-bouillon tube, and so on. These were then poured upon large surfaces and allowed to solidify. The results were entirely satisfactory. On the gelatin plates from the original tube, as was expected, the colonies were too numerous to be of any use; on the plates made from the first dilution they were much fewer in number, but still they were usually too numerous and too closely packed to permit of characteristic growth; but on the second dilution they were, as a rule, fewer in number and widely separated, so that the individuals of each species were in no way prevented by the proximity of its neighbors from growing in its own typical way. There was then no difficulty in picking out the colonies resulting from the growth of the different individual bacteria.

Such, then, are the principles upon which Koch's method for the isolation of bacteria by means of solid media is based.

The fundamental part of the media employed is the bouillon, which contains all the elements necessary for the nutrition of most bacteria, the gelatin being employed simply for the purpose of rendering the bouillon solid. The medium on which the organisms are growing is, therefore, simply solidified bouillon, or beef tea.

In practice, two forms of gelatin are employed—the one an animal or bone gelatin, the ordinary table gelatin of good quality; and the other a vegetable gelatin, known as agar-agar, or Japanese gelatin, which is obtained from a group of algæ growing in the sea along the coast of Japan, where it is employed as an article of diet by the natives.

Aside from these differences in origin of the two forms of gelatin employed, their behavior toward heat and toward bacteria renders them of different application in the bacteriological work. The animal gelatin liquefies at a much lower temperature, and likewise solidifies at a very much lower temperature, than does the agar-agar. Ordinary gelatin liquefies at about 24° C., and becomes solid at from 8°–10° C. It may be employed for those organisms which do not require a higher temperature for their development than 22° C. Agar-agar, on the other hand, does not liquefy until the temperature has reached about

98°–99° C. It remains fluid ordinarily until the temperature has fallen to 38°–39° C., when it rapidly solidifies. For our purposes, only that form of agar-agar can be used which remains fluid at from 38°–40° C. Agar-agar which remains fluid only at a temperature above this point would be too hot, when in a fluid state, for use; many of the organisms which would be introduced into it would either be destroyed or checked in their development by so high a temperature. Agar-agar, therefore, is for use in those cases in which the cultivation must be conducted at a temperature above that at which gelatin remains solid.

In addition to the differences toward temperature, the relations of these two gelatins to bacteria are different. Many bacteria bring about alterations in gelatin which cause it to become liquid (probably a process of peptonization), in which state it remains. There are no known organisms which bring about such a change in the agar-agar.

As a rule, the colony-formations seen upon gelatine are much more characteristic than those which develop on agar-agar, and for this reason gelatin is to be preferred when circumstances will permit. Both gelatin and agar-agar may be used in the preparation of plates and Esmarch tubes, subsequently to be described.

CHAPTER VI.

Preparation of media—Bouillon, gelatin, agar-agar, potato, blood-serum, etc.

As has been stated, the fundamental part of our culture media is beef tea, or bouillon.

BOUILLON.—The formula of Koch for the preparation of this medium has undergone many modifications to meet special cases, but for general use his original formula is still retained. It is as follows: Five hundred grammes of finely-chopped lean beef, free from fat and tendons, is to be soaked in one litre of water for twenty-four hours. During this time it is to remain in the ice-chest or to be kept at a low temperature. It is then to be strained through a coarse towel and pressed until a litre of fluid is obtained. To this is to be added ten grammes (1.0 per cent.) of dried peptone and five grammes (0.5 per cent.) of common salt (NaCl). It is then to be rendered exactly neutral or very slightly alkaline, with a few drops of saturated soda solution. The flask containing the mixture is then to be placed either in the steam sterilizer or on a water-bath, or over a free flame, and kept at the boiling-point until all the albumin is coagulated, and the fluid portion is of a clear, pale, straw-color. It is then filtered through a folded paper filter, and sterilized in the steam sterilizer by the fractional method. Certain of the modifications of this method are of sufficient value to justify mention. Most important is the neutralization. Ordinarily, this is accomplished with the saturated soda solution, and the reaction is detected with the ordinary red and blue litmus paper.

Soda solution is not so good as a strong solution of caustic soda or potash, because the carbonic acid liberated from the sodium carbonate is frequently seen to give rise to a confusing temporary acid reaction which disappears on heating. To obviate this, Schultz (*Centralbl. f. Bact. u. Parasitenkunde*, Bd. x., Nos. 2 and 3, 1891) recommends exact titration with a solution of caustic soda. For this purpose a 4 per cent. solution of caustic soda is prepared. From this a 0.4 per cent. solution is made, and with it the titration is practised. After the bouillon has been deprived of all coagulable albumin and blood coloring matter by boiling and filtration, and has cooled down to the temperature of the air, its whole volume is exactly measured.

From it a sample of exactly 5 or 10 c.c. is then taken, and to it a few drops of one of the indicators commonly employed in analytical work is added. Schultz recommends 1 drop of phenolphtalein solution (1 gramme phenolphtalein in 300 c.c. of alcohol) to 1 c.c. of bouillon. The beaker containing the sample is placed upon white paper, and the dilute caustic soda solution is then allowed to drop into it, very slowly, from a burette, until there appears a very delicate rose color, which indicates the beginning of alkaline reaction. A second sample of the bouillon is treated in the same way. If the amounts of soda solution required for each sample deviate but very slightly or not at all the one from the other, the mean of these amounts is taken as the amount of the soda solution necessary to neutralize the quantity of bouillon employed. If 10 c.c.

of bouillon were employed, then, for the whole amount of 1 litre, just 100 times as much, minus that for the two samples used in titration, will be needed. For example: To neutralize 10 c.c. of bouillon, 2 c.c. of the diluted (0.4 per cent.) caustic soda solution were employed. For the remaining 980 c.c. of the litre of bouillon, then, 200 c.c. (—4 c.c., the amount employed for the two samples of 10 c.c. each of bouillon) is needed of the 0.4 per cent. solution, or one-tenth of this amount of the 4 per cent. solution.

For the neutralization of the whole bulk of the bouillon it is better to employ the strong alkaline solution, as by its use the volume is not increased to so great an extent as when the dilute solution is used.

It is evident that this method is much more exact than that ordinarily employed, but at the same time it must be remembered that for its success it requires exactness in the measurement of the volumes and the preparation of the dilutions. To obviate error, it is better to employ this method when the solutions are all cool and of nearly the same temperature, so that rapid fluctuations in temperature, and consequent alterations in volume, will not materially interfere with the accuracy of the results.

This method of neutralization, which is employed by Schultz, is to be recommended for those experiments in which slight inaccuracies in the reaction of the media play an important part.

For the ordinary purposes of the beginner, however, results quite satisfactory in their nature may be obtained by the employment of the saturated soda solution for neutralization and the litmus paper as the indicator. For some time, however, it has been our practice to employ the yellow curcuma paper for the detection of alkalinity rather than the red litmus paper.

Not infrequently the filtered bouillon, neutralized and sterilized, will be seen to contain a fine, flocculent precipitate. This may be due either to excess of alkalinity or to incomplete precipitation of the albumin. The former may be corrected with dilute acetic or hydrochloric acid, and the bouillon again boiled, filtered, and sterilized; or, if due to the latter cause, subsequent boiling and filtration usually results in ridding the bouillon of the precipitate.

NUTRIENT GELATIN.—For the preparation of gelatin the bouillon is first prepared in exactly the same way as has just been described, except that the neutralization takes place after the gelatin has been completely dissolved, which occurs very rapidly in hot bouillon. The reaction of the gelatin as it comes from the manufactories is usually quite acid, so that a much larger amount of alkali is needed for its neutralization than for other media. The gelatin is added in the proportion of from 10 to 12 per cent. The complete solution of the gelatin may be accomplished either over the water-bath, in the steam sterilizer, or over a free flame. If the latter method is practised, care must be given that the mixture is constantly stirred to prevent burning at the bottom and consequent breaking of the flask, if a flask is employed.

For some time it has been our practice to use, for the purpose of making both gelatin and agar, enamelled iron saucepans instead of glass flasks; by this means the free flame may be employed without danger of breaking the vessel, and, with a little care, without fear of burning the media. Under any conditions it is better to protect the bottom of the vessel from the direct action of the flame by the interposition of several layers of wire gauze or a thin sheet of asbestos-board.

When the gelatin is completely melted, it may be filtered through a folded paper filter on an ordinary funnel; if the solution is perfect, this should be very quickly accomplished.

The employment of the hot-water funnel, so often recommended, has been dispensed with in this work to a very large extent, as we know that, if the solution of the gelatin is complete, filtration is so rapid as not to necessitate the use of an apparatus for maintaining the high temperature. The temperature at which the hot-water funnel retains the gelatin is so high that evaporation and condensation rapidly occur, and in consequence the filtration is, as a rule, retarded. The filtration is frequently done in the steam sterilizer, but this is unnecessary if the gelatin is quite dissolved. At the ordinary temperature of the room and by the means commonly employed for the filtration of other substances, both gelatin and agar-agar may be rapidly filtered if they are completely dissolved.

It not infrequently occurs that, even under the most careful treatment, the filtered gelatin is not perfectly transparent (the condition in which it must exist, otherwise it is useless), and clarification becomes necessary. For this purpose the mass must be redissolved, and when at a temperature between 60° C. and 70° C., the whites of two eggs, which have been beaten up with about 50 c.c. of water, are added. The whole is then thoroughly mixed together and again brought to the boiling-point, and kept at this point until coagulation of the albumin occurs. It is better not to break up the large masses of coagulated albumin if it can be avoided, as when broken up into fine flakes they clog the filter and render filtration very difficult.

The practice sometimes recommended of removing these albuminous masses by first filtering the gelatin through a cloth, and then finally through paper, is not only superfluous, but in most instances renders the process of filtration much more difficult, because of the disintegration of these masses into the finer particles, which have the effect just mentioned.

Under no circumstances is a filter to be used for these purposes without first having been moistened with water. If this is not done, the pores of the paper, which are relatively large when in a dry state, when moistened by the gelatin not only diminish in size, but in contracting are often entirely occluded by the finer albuminous flakes which become fixed within them. In this way the filter may become almost entirely occluded. The preliminary moistening with water causes the diminution of the size of the pores to such an extent that the finer particles of the precipitate now rest *on* the surface of the paper, instead of becoming fixed *in its meshes*.

During boiling it is well to filter from time to time a few cubic centimetres of the gelatin into a test-tube and boil it over a free flame for a minute or so; in this way one can detect if all the albumin has been coagulated and when the solution is ready for filtration.

Gelatin should not, as a rule, be boiled over ten or fifteen minutes at one time, or left in the steam sterilizer for more than thirty to forty-five minutes, otherwise its property of solidifying is materially diminished.

As soon as the gelatin is complete, whether it is

retained in the flask into which it has been filtered or decanted off into sterilized test-tubes, it should be sterilized in the steam sterilizer on three successive days, for fifteen minutes each day—the mouth of the flask or the test-tubes containing it having been previously closed with cotton plugs.

NUTRIENT AGAR-AGAR.—The preparation of the nutrient agar-agar by the beginner is, as a rule, a somewhat tedious and time-taking experience. This is owing mainly to lack of patience and failure to adhere strictly to the rules laid down for the preparation of this medium. Many methods are recommended for its preparation; almost every worker has some slight modification of his own.

The method which has given the best results in our hands, and from which there are no grounds for deviating, is as follows:

Prepare the bouillon in the usual way. Agar-agar reacts neutral, so that the bouillon may be neutralized before the agar is added. Then add finely-chopped agar in the proportion of 1 to 1.5 per cent. Place the mixture in a porcelain-lined iron vessel and make a mark on the sides of the vessel at which the level of the fluid stands, add about 250 c.c. of water and allow the mass to boil slowly, occasionally stirring, over a free flame for three or four hours. Care must be given that it does not boil over the sides of the vessel. From time to time observe if the fluid has fallen below the mark of its original level; if it has, add water until its original volume is restored. At the end of the time given remove the flame and place the vessel containing the mixture in a large dish of cold water; stir the agar continously until it has cooled down to about 68°–70° C., and then add the whites of two eggs which have been beaten up in about 50 c.c. of water. Mix this carefully throughout the agar, and allow the mass to boil slowly for about one-half hour, observing all the while the level of the fluid. It is necessary to reduce the temperature of the mass to the extent given, 68°–70° C., otherwise the coagulation of the albumin will occur in lumps and masses as soon as it is added, and its clearing action will not be homogeneous. The process is a purely mechanical one—the finer particles, which would otherwise pass through the pores of the filter, being taken up by the albumin as it coagulates and retained in the coagula.

At the end of one-half hour the boiling mass may be easily and quickly filtered through a heavy, folded paper filter at the room temperature, and, as a rule, the filtrate is as clear and as transparent as agar-agar usually appears. If the mixture is positively alkaline, it is not only cloudy, but it filters with difficulty; if it is acid, it is usually quite clear; but, as Schultz has pointed out, it loses at the same time some of its gelatinizing properties. The bouillon should always be neutralized before the agar-agar is added to it, for the bouillon, which is normally acid, from the acid of the meat, robs the agar, under the influence of heat, of some of its gelatinizing powers; this cannot be regained by subsequent neutralization.

Another method by which the agar-agar can easily and quickly be melted, is by steam under pressure. If the flask containing the mixture of bouillon and agar be kept in the digestor or autoclav, with the steam under a pressure of one atmosphere, as shown by the gauge, for from twenty to thirty minutes, the agar-agar will be found at the end of this time completely melted, and filtration may then be accomplished with but little difficulty.

If glycerin is to be added to the agar-agar, it is done after filtration and before sterilization. The nutritive properties of the media for certain organisms, particularly the tubercle bacillus, is improved by the addition of glycerin in the proportion of 5 to 7 per cent.

If after filtration a fine flocculent precipitate is seen, look to the reaction of the medium. If it is quite alkaline, neutralize, boil, and filter again. If the reaction is neutral or only very slightly acid, dissolve and clarify again with egg albumin by the method given.

The most important point in all the media, aside from the correct proportion of the ingredients, is their reaction. They must be neutral or very slightly alkaline. But few organisms develop well on media of an acid reaction. In all of the above media the meat extracts now on the market may occasionally be substituted for the meat itself in preparing the bouillon. In this case the preparation known as Liebig's Meat Extract may be employed in the proportion of from three to five grammes to the litre of water.

PREPARATION OF POTATOES.—Potatoes are prepared for use in two ways:

1. They are taken as they come to the market—old potatoes being usually recommended, and carefully scrubbed under the water-tap with a stiff brush until all adherent dirt has been removed; "the eyes" and all discolored or decayed parts are carefully removed with a pointed knife. They are then to be placed in a solution of corrosive sublimate of the strength of 1:1000 and allowed to remain there for twenty minutes; at the end of this time, without rinsing off the sublimate, they are placed into a covered tin bucket with a perforated bottom and sterilized in the steam sterilizer for forty-

five minutes. On the second and third days the sterilization is repeated for fifteen to twenty minutes each day. They must not be removed from the sterilizing bucket until sterilization is complete. At the end of this time they are ready for use. When prepared in this way, they are usually intended to be cut into two halves, and the cultivation of the organisms is to be conducted upon the flat surfaces of the sections.

This method requires some care to prevent contamination during manipulation. The hand which is to take up the potato from the bucket, which until now has remained covered, is first disinfected in the sublimate solution for ten minutes, the potato is then taken up between the thumb and index finger, and severed into two by a knife which has just been sterilized in the free flame until it is quite hot. The blade of the knife is passed not quite through the potato, but nearly so. A large glass culture-dish for the reception of the two halves of the potato having been disinfected for twenty minutes with 1 : 1000 sublimate solution and then drained of all the adherent solution, is at hand ready for the bits of potato; the cover is removed, and by twisting the knife gently the two halves of the potato may be caused to fall apart in the dish and usually to fall upon their convex surfaces, leaving the flat sections uppermost. The cover is placed upon the dish and the potatoes are ready for inoculation.

2. *Preparation of potatoes for test-tube cultures.* If the potatoes are to be employed for test-tube cultures, one simply scrubs off the coarser particles of dirt with water and a brush, and with a cork-borer punches out cylindrical bits of potato which will fit loosely into the test-tubes to be used. On each bit of potato is then

to be cut a slanting surface running diagonally from about the junction of the first and second third of the cylinder to the diagonally opposite end. These cylinders of potato are now to be left in running water over night, otherwise they are very much discolored by the sterilization to which they are to be subjected. At the end of this time they are placed into previously prepared test-tubes, one piece in each tube, with the slanting surface up, the cotton plugs of the tubes replaced and they are then to be sterilized in the steam for forty-five minutes. On the second or third day they are to be sterilized for fifteen to twenty minutes each day.

FIG. 6.

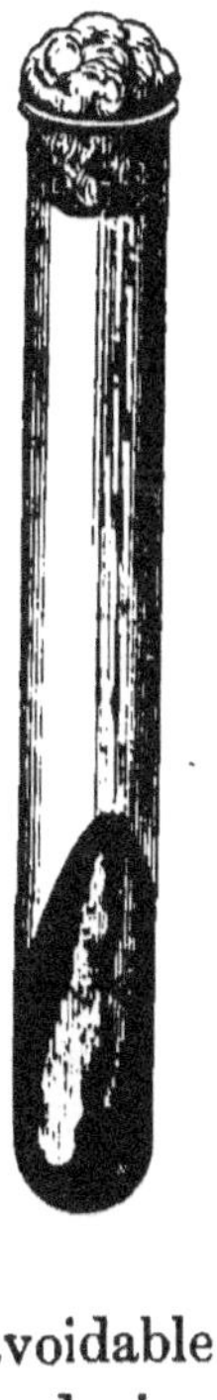

The entire sterilization may be accomplished in the autoclav with the steam under a pressure of one atmosphere, by a single exposure of twenty to twenty-five minutes. When finished they have the appearance seen in Fig. 6.

Care must be given to the sterilization of potatoes, because they always have adhering to them the organisms commonly found in the ground, the spores of which are among the most resistant of all known organisms. The so-called "potato bacillus" is one of this group; it is an organism which not infrequently is more or less of an obstacle to the work of the beginner.

BLOOD-SERUM. — Blood-serum requires special care in its preparation; it is desirable under all conditions to reduce the unavoidable contamination which to a certain extent occurs during the manipulation, to its minimum degree.

It is possible to collect serum from small animals and

in small quantities under such precautions that it is perhaps not contaminated, but ordinarily for laboratory purposes a larger quantity is needed, so that the slaughter-houses form the sources from which it is usually obtained, and here a certain amount of contamination is unavoidable, though its degree may be limited by proper precaution. The animal from which the blood is to be collected should be drawn up to the ceiling by the hind legs, the head should be held well back, and with one pass of a very sharp knife the throat should be completely cut through. The blood which will be spurting from the severed vessels should be collected in large glass jars which have been previously cleaned, disinfected, and all traces of the disinfectant removed with alcohol and finally ether. The latter evaporates very quickly and leaves the jar quite dry. The jars should be provided with covers which close hermetically—these too should be carefully disinfected. The best form of glass vessels for the purpose are the large glass museum jars of about one gallon capacity, which close by a cover which can be tightly screwed down upon a rubber joint. From two such jarfuls of blood one can recover quite a large quantity of serum, ordinarily from 500–700 c.c. The jars having been filled with blood, their covers are placed loosely upon them and they are allowed to stand for about fifteen minutes until clotting has begun. At the end of this time a clean glass rod is passed around the edges of the surface of the clot to break up any adhesions to the wall of the jar that might have formed, and which would prevent the sinking of the clot to the bottom. The covers are then tightly replaced, and with as little agitation as possible the jars are placed in an ice-chest, where they remain for twenty-four to forty-eight hours. The temperature should, however, not be low enough to prevent coagulation, but should be sufficiently low to interfere with the development of any living organisms that may be present. The temperature of the ordinary domestic refrigerator is sufficient for the purpose. After twenty-four to forty-eight hours the clot will have become firm, and will be seen at the bottom of the jar. Above it is a quantity of dark straw-colored serum. The serum may then be drawn off with a sterilized pipette and placed in tall cylinders which have previously been plugged with cotton wadding and sterilized. After treating all the serum in this way, care having been taken to get as little of the coloring matter of the blood as possible, it may be placed again in the ice-chest for twenty-four hours during which time the corpuscular elements will sink to the bottom, leaving the supernatant fluid quite clear. This may then be pipetted off, either into sterilized test-tubes, about 8 c.c. to each tube, or into small sterilized flasks of about 100 c.c. capacity. It is then to be sterilized by the intermittent method *at low temperatures*, viz., for one hour on each of five consecutive days at a temperature of 68°–70° C. During the intervening days it is to be kept at the room temperature to permit of the development of any spores that may be present into their vegetative forms, in which condition they are killed by an hour's exposure to the temperature of 70° C.

At the end of this time the serum in the tubes may either be retained as fluid serum or solidified at between 76°–80° C. In solidifying the serum the tubes should be placed in an inclined position so that as great a surface as possible may be given to the serum. The process of solidification requires constant attention if good results are to be obtained, *i. e.*, if a translucent, solid medium is to result. If the old, small form of apparatus is employed (Fig. 7), then the solidification can be accomplished in a shorter time than if the larger forms, which are now frequently employed, are used. No definite rule for the time that will be required can be laid down, for this is not constant. If the small solidifying apparatus is used, very good results may be obtained in about two hours at 78° C. It frequently requires a longer time at a higher temperature than has been mentioned. This is especially the case with Löffler's serum mixture.

Fig. 7.

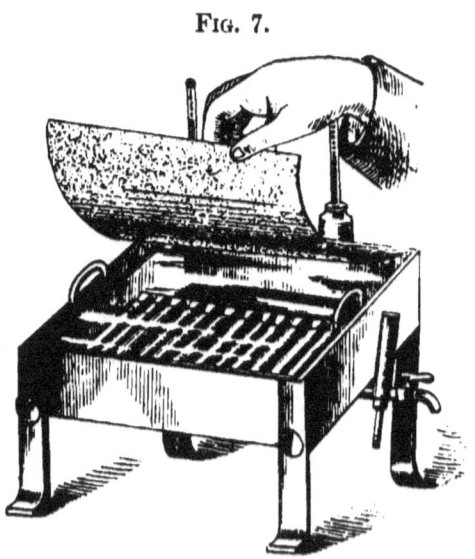

The best results are obtained when a low temperature is employed for a long time. Under any circumstances the tubes must be observed from time to time through the glass door or cover with which the solidifying oven is provided, and each time the oven should be slightly jarred with the hand to see if solidification, as indicated by the disappearance of tremors from the serum, is beginning. If the temperature gets too high, or the exposure is too long, an opaque medium results. The temperature to be observed is that of the air inside the chamber, and also that of the water surrounding it. The latter is usually a degree or two higher than the former. The tubes should not rest directly upon the heated bottom or against the heated sides of the chamber, but should lie upon racks of wood or wire, and be protected from the sides by a wire screen of gauze; in this way the tubes are all exposed to about the same temperature. The thermometer which indicates the temperature inside the chamber should not touch the surfaces but should either be suspended free from above through a cork in the top of the apparatus, if the large form of apparatus is used, or should lie upon a rack of cork or wood, its bulb being free and a little lower than the other extremity, if the small, old-fashioned apparatus of Koch is employed. The latter form is preferable, as it is more easily managed.

When solidification is complete, the tubes are to be retained in the erect position and, unless they are intended for immediate use, must be prevented from drying. The superfluous ends of the cotton plugs should be burned off, and the mouths of the tubes should then be covered by sterilized rubber caps. Even with the greatest care, it not uncommonly happens that one or two of the lot of tubes thus prepared and protected will become contaminated. This is usually due to spores of moulds that have fallen into the rubber caps or on the cotton plugs during manipulation, and, finding no means of outward growth, have thrown their hyphen downward through the cotton into the tube, and their spores have fallen upon the surface of the serum and gone on to develop.

SPECIAL MEDIA.—The media just described—bouillon, nutrient gelatin, nutrient agar-agar, potato, and blood-serum—are those in general use in the laboratory for purposes of isolation and study of the ordinary forms of bacteria. For the finer points of differentiation special media have been suggested; a few of them will be mentioned.

Milk. Fresh milk should be allowed to stand over night in the ice-chest, the cream then removed, and the remainder of the milk pipetted into test-tubes, about 8 c.c. to each tube, and sterilized by the intermittent process, at the temperature of steam, for three successive days.

The cream is best separated from the milk by the use of a cylindrical vessel with stop-cock at the bottom, by means of which the milk, devoid of cream, may be drawn off. A Chevallier creamometer with stop-cock at the bottom serves the purpose very well. It should be covered while standing.

Milk may be used as a culture medium without any addition to it, or, before sterilizing, a few drops of litmus tincture may be added, just enough to give it a pale blue color. By this means it may be seen that different organisms bring about different reactions in the medium; some producing alkalies which cause the blue color to be intensified, others producing acids which change it to red, while others bring about neither of these changes.

Milk may also be employed as a solid culture medium by the addition to it of gelatin or agar-agar in the proportions given for the preparation of the ordinary nutrient gelatin or agar-agar. It has, however, in this form the disadvantage of not being transparent, and can therefore best be used for the study of those organisms which grow upon the surface of the medium without causing liquefaction.

Nutrient gelatin and agar-agar can also be prepared from neutral milk whey, obtained from milk by precipitation of the casein.

Dunham's solution and peptone-rosalic-acid solution. Peptone solution, to which rosalic acid has been added, also serves very well for the detection of alterations in reaction. The peptone solution of Dunham is the form that we have usually employed. It consists of

Distilled water	100 parts.
Dried peptone	1 part.
Sodium chloride	0.5 "

and 4 c.c. of the following solution :

Rosalic acid (coralline)	0.5 gramme.
Alcohol (80 per cent.)	100 c.c.

This is to be boiled, filtered, and decanted into clean, sterilized test-tubes, about 8 to 10 c.c. to each tube. The tubes are then to be sterilized in the usual way by steam. When sterilization is completed and the tubes cooled, the solution will be of a very pale rose color, which disappears entirely under the action of acids, and becomes much more intense when alkalies are produced. We have used this solution for some time for the study of the reactions produced by different organisms, and find it a valuable addition to our means of differentiation of bacteria.

Löffler's blood-serum mixture. Löffler's blood-serum mixture consists of one part of neutral meat-infusion bouillon containing 1 per cent. of grape-sugar, and three parts of blood-serum. This mixture is placed in test-tubes, sterilized, and solidified in exactly the way given for blood serum.

Guarniari's agar-gelatin:

Meat-infusion	950 c.c.
Sodium chloride	5 grammes.
Peptone	25–30 "
Gelatin	40–60 "
Agar-agar	3–4 "
Water	50 c.c.

The point in the preparation of this medium is its reaction, which should be exactly neutral.

The list of special media is too great to be given in a work of this size. Their description must be seen in the original. Those which have been given above will suffice for obtaining a clear understanding of the principles of the work.

NOTE.—The term "meat-infusion" always implies a watery extract of meat made by mixing 500 grammes of finely-chopped lean meat and 1 litre of water together, and allowing them to stand in a cool place for twenty-four hours. At the end of this time the fluid portion is strained off through a coarse towel. This represents the infusion.

CHAPTER VII.

Preparation of the tubes, flasks, etc., in which the media are to be preserved.

WHILE the media are in course of preparation it is well to get the test-tubes and flasks ready for their reception. It is essential that the tubes for this purpose should be as clean as it is possible to make them. For this purpose it is advisable that both new tubes and those which have previously been used should be boiled for some time, about thirty to forty-five minutes, in a strong solution of common soda, about a 4 or 6 per cent. solution; it is not necessary to be exact as to the strength, but it should not be weaker than this. At the end of this time they are to be carefully swabbed out with a cylindrical bristle brush, preferably one having a reed handle (Fig. 8), as those with wire handles are apt to break

FIG. 8.

through the bottoms of the tubes. All trace of adherent material should be carefully removed. When the tubes are quite clean they may be rinsed in a warm solution of commercial hydrochloric acid of the strength of about 1 per cent. This is to remove the alkali. They are then to be thoroughly rinsed in clear, running water, and stood top down until the water has drained from them. When dry they are to be plugged with raw cotton. The plugging with the cotton requires a little practice before it can be properly done. The cotton should be introduced into the mouths of the tubes in such a way that no cracks or creases exist, but should fill them quite regularly all around. The plugs should be neither too tight nor too loose, the regular rule being that when in position the plug should fit tight enough to just sustain the weight of the tube into which it is placed when held up by the portion which projects from and overhangs the mouth of the tube. The tubes thus plugged with cotton are now to be placed upright in a wire basket and heated for one hour in the hot-air sterilizer at a temperature of about 150° C. A very good rule for this process of sterilizing is to observe the tubes from time to time, and as soon as the cotton has become a very light brown color, not deeper than a dark-cream tint, to consider sterilization complete. The tubes are then removed and allowed to cool down.

The cotton used for this purpose should be the ordinary cotton batting of the shops, and not absorbent cotton, the latter becomes too tightly packed, and is, moreover, much too expensive for this purpose.

Care should be taken not to burn the cotton, otherwise the tubes will become coated with a dark-colored oily deposit which renders them unfit for use, and they will have to be cleaned again.

FILLING THE TUBES.—When the tubes are cold they may be filled. This is best accomplished by the use of a spherical form of funnel, such as is shown in Fig. 9. The liquefied medium is poured into this funnel, which has been carefully washed, and by pressing the pinch-cock with which the funnel is provided, the

FILLING THE TUBES. 79

desired amount of material (5–10 c.c.) may be allowed to flow into the tubes held under its opening.

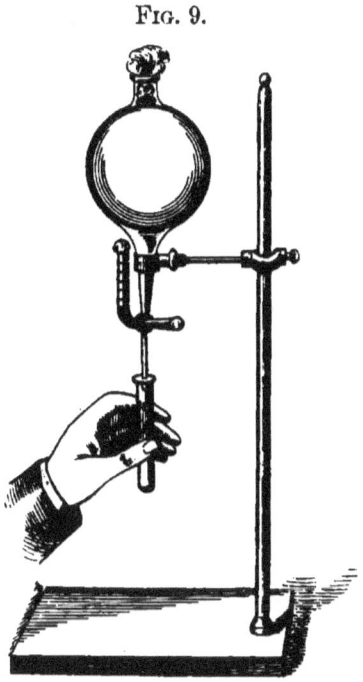

Fig. 9.

It is not necessary to sterilize the funnel, for the medium is to be subjected to this process as soon as it is in the test-tubes.

Care should be given that none of the medium is dropped upon the mouth of the test-tube, otherwise the cotton plugs become adherent to the tube and are not only difficult to remove, but present a very untidy appearance, and interfere, indeed, with the proper manipulations.

As soon as the tubes have been filled they are to be sterilized in the steam sterilizer for fifteen minutes on each of three successive days. During the intervening days they may be kept at the ordinary room temperature.

When sterilization is complete, and the medium in the tubes is still liquid, some of them may be placed in a slanting position, at an angle of about ten degrees with the surface on which they rest, and the medium allowed to solidify in this position. These are for the so-called slant cultures. The balance may solidify in the erect position; these serve for the plate cultures.

For Esmarch tubes not more than 5 c.c. of material should be placed in each tube, as more than this renders the rolling difficult and irregular.

CHAPTER VIII.

Technique of making plates—Esmarch tubes, Petri plates, etc.

PLATES.—The plate method can be practised with both agar-agar and gelatin. It cannot be practised with blood-serum, because the serum, when once solidified, cannot be again liquefied.

Plates are usually referred to as "a set." This term implies three individual plates each representing the mixture of organisms in a higher stage of dilution. The first plate is known usually as "the original," or "plate 1," the first dilution from this as "plate 2," and the second as "plate 3."

In the preparation of a set of plates the following are the steps to be observed :

Three tubes, each containing from 7 to 9 c.c. of gelatin or agar-agar, are placed in the water-bath until the medium has become liquid. If agar-agar is employed, this is accomplished at the boiling-point of water; if gelatin is used, a much lower temperature suffices ($35°$–$40°$ C.). When liquefaction is complete the temperature of the water, in the case of agar-agar, must be reduced to $41°$–$42°$ C., at which temperature the agar-agar remains liquid and the organisms may be introduced into it without fear of destroying their vitality. The medium being now liquid and of the proper temperature, a very small portion of the mixture of organisms to be studied is taken up with a sterilized, looped platinum wire, an "oese" as it is called, Fig. 10. This is nothing more than a piece of platinum wire of about 5 c.m. long, twisted into a small loop at one end and fused into a bit of glass rod, which acts as a handle, at the other extremity. This "oese" is one of the most useful of bacteriological instruments, as there is hardly a manipulation in the work into which it does not enter. Under no conditions is it to be

FIG. 10.

employed without having been passed through the gas-flame until quite hot; this is for the purpose of sterilization. One should form a habit of never taking up one of these "oeses," or platinum-wire needles, as they are also called, for they are both looped and curved or straight, without passing it through the flame, and the sooner the beginner learns to do this as a matter of reflex, the sooner does he rid himself of one of the possible sources of error in his work. It must be remembered, though, that the "oese" should not be used when hot, otherwise the organisms taken up with it are killed by the high temperature; after sterilizing it in the flame one waits for a few seconds before using it.

The bit of material under consideration is transferred with the sterilized "oese" into tube No. 1, "the original," where it is carefully disintegrated by gently rubbing it against the sides of the tube. The more carefully this is done the more homogeneous will be the

TECENIQUE OF MAKING PLATES. 83

distribution of the organisms and the better the results. The "oese" is then again sterilized, and three of its loopfuls are passed, without touching the sides of the tube, from "the original" into tube No. 2, where they are carefully mixed. Again the "oese" is sterilized and again three dips are made from tube 2 into tube 3. This completes the dilution. The "oese" is now sterilized before laying it aside.

FIG. 11.

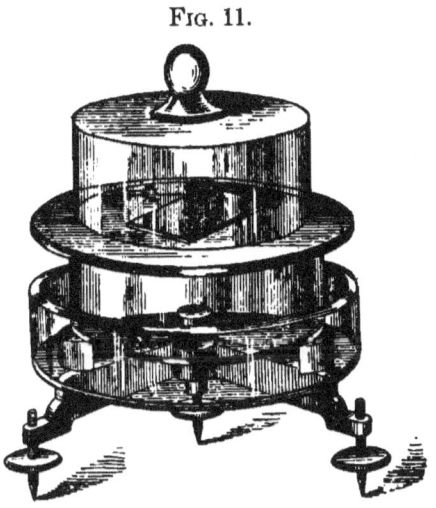

During this manipulation, which must be done quickly if agar-agar is employed, the temperature of the water in the bath in which the tubes stand should never get lower than 39° C., and never higher than 43° C. If it falls too low, below 38° C., the agar gelatinizes, and can only be redissolved by a temperature which would be destructive to the organisms which may have been introduced into the tubes. This is not of so much moment with gelatin, as it may readily be redissolved at a temperature not detrimental to the organisms with which the tubes may have been inoculated

THE COOLING-STAGE AND LEVELLING TRIPOD.—While the medium of which the plates are to be made is melting, it is well to arrange the cooling-stage (Fig. 11) upon which it is to be subsequently solidified.

This stage consists of a glass dish filled with ice-water and covered with a ground-glass plate, which in turn has a dome-shaped cover. The dish rests upon a tripod which can be brought to an exact level, as indicated by the spirit-level, by raising or lowering its legs by means of screws, with which they are provided. Three stages are usually employed. When ready for use they should be exactly level.

THE GLASS PLATES.—On the stages are to be placed the glass plates upon which the liquefied gelatin or agar-agar is to be poured and allowed to solidify. It is

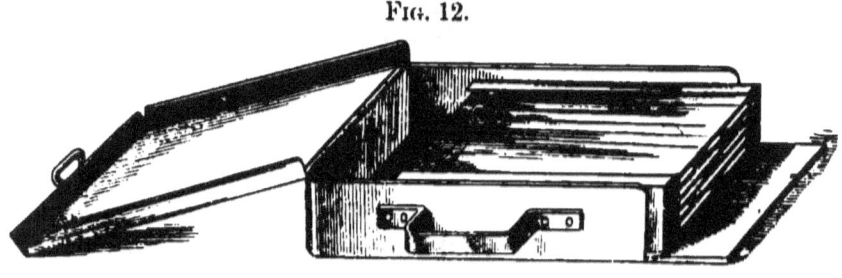

FIG. 12.

therefore necessary that the plates should not only be sterile when placed upon the stages, but should be carefully protected by a cover against dust and bacteria from outside sources during manipulation.

A number of plates at a time are usually sterilized in the dry sterilizer at a temperature of 150° to 180° C. for one hour. During sterilization and until used they are retained in an iron box (Fig. 12), which is especially designed for the purpose.

They should never be placed upon the stage until cold, otherwise they crack.

When the plates which have been placed upon the stages are quite cold, the melted gelatin or agar-agar in the tubes which represent the three dilutions should be poured upon them, each tube being emptied upon a separate plate. If the medium is quite fluid it spreads over the surface of the plates in a thin even layer. Sometimes it may be more evenly spread as it flows from the tube by the aid of a sterilized glass rod.

As the contents of each tube is emptied upon a plate the cover of the cooling-stage is quickly replaced and the plate allowed to stand until the gelatin or agar-agar is quite solid. This takes longer with gelatin than with agar. When quite solid they are placed upon little glass benches (Fig. 13), and each bench is

FIG. 13.

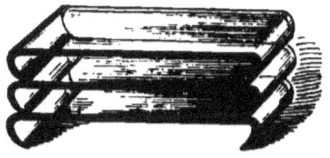

labelled with the number of the plate in the series of dilutions. The benches, with the plates upon them, are then piled one above the other in a glass dish, the so-called "culture-dish," in which the plates are to be kept during the growth of the bacteria. The benches are sterilized before using, in the way given for the plates.

CULTURE-DISH.—This dish, which is about 22 cm. in diameter and has vertical sides of about 6 cm. in height, is provided with a cover of exactly the same design, but of a little larger diameter. This cover, when placed upon the dish containing the plates, fits over it and prevents the access of dust. Prior to using, the dish and cover should have been disinfected for one-half hour with 1:1000 sublimate, and then all the sublimate solution allowed to drain from it.

Into the bottom of this dish is sometimes placed a disc of sterilized filter-paper moistened with sterilized water, which serves to prevent the drying of the plates. This, however, is not necessary.

If agar-agar is employed, the dish and its contents may be placed at a temperature of 37°–38° C.; if gelatin, the temperature at which the plates are now to be kept should not be over 22° C., otherwise the gelatin becomes liquefied and the plates are rendered useless.

When development has occurred, the object of the dilution will easily be seen, and the different species of bacteria in the mixture will be recognized by differences in the character of the colonies growing from them.

This, in short, is the plate method of Koch for the separation of the individual species contained in a mixture of bacteria. Many modifications of this method exist; all, however, are based upon the same principles. The modifications have for their object the accomplishment of the same end, but with a smaller armamentarium of apparatus.

PETRI'S MODIFICATION OF THE PLATE METHOD.—The modification which approaches nearest to the original method, and at the same time lessens very materially the number of steps in the process, is that suggested by Petri. It consists in substituting for the plates small, round, double glass dishes, which have about the same surface-

ESMARCH'S TUBES. 87

area as the plates. The liquid medium may be poured directly into these little dishes without their being exactly level. Each dish acts as a plate. Their covers are then to be replaced, and they are set aside for observation. In all other respects the steps are the same as those given for Koch's original method. Petri's dishes are flat, double dishes of glass (Fig. 14). They are of about 8 cm. in

FIG. 14.

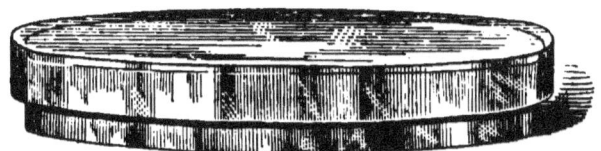

diameter and about 1.5 to 2 cm. in height, the walls being vertical. They may readily be sterilized either by the hot-air or steam methods of sterilization. They are very useful for this work, as they do away with the necessity for the cooling-stage and levelling tripods, though in warm weather the cooling-stage may be used to hasten the solidification of gelatin.

ESMARCH'S TUBES.—The modification of Koch's method which insures the greatest security from contamination by outside organisms and requires the smallest supply of apparatus, is that suggested by v. Esmarch. It differs from the other methods thus: The dilutions having been prepared in tubes containing a smaller amount of medium than usual—as a rule not more than 5 to 6 c.c.—are, instead of being poured out upon plates or into dishes, spread over the inner surface of the tube containing them, and without removing the cotton plugs are caused to solidify in this position. The tubes then present a thin cylindrical lining of gelatin or agar-agar, upon which the colonies develop. In all other respects the conditions for the growth of the organisms are the same as in flat plates.

Esmarch directs that after completion of the dilutions the tops of the cotton plugs in the tubes should be cut off flush with the mouth of the test-tube and a rubber cap be placed over this. They are then to be held in the horizontal position and twisted between the fingers upon their long axes under ice-water. The gelatin becomes solidified thereby and adheres to the sides of the tube. When the gelatin is quite hard the tubes are removed from the water, wiped dry, the rubber caps removed, and they are set aside for observation.

Fig. 15.

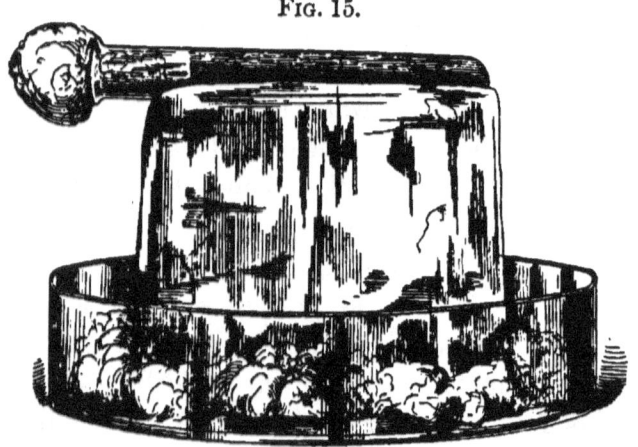

For some time past we have deviated from the directions given by v. Esmarch for this part of his method. Instead of rolling the tubes under ice-water, we roll them upon a block of ice (Fig. 15). In this method a small block of ice only is needed. It is arranged nearly level, and is held in position by being placed in a dish upon cloths. A horizontal groove is melted in the surface of the ice with a test-tube of hot water. The tubes to be rolled are then held in an almost, *not quite*, horizontal position and twisted between the fingers until the sides are moistened by the contents to within about 1 cm. of the cotton plug, care being taken that the gelatin *does not touch* the cotton; otherwise the latter becomes adherent to the sides of the tube and is difficult to remove. The tube is then placed in the groove in the ice and rolled, no rubber cap or cutting off of the cotton plug being necessary.

The advantages of this process over that followed by v. Esmarch are that it requires less time, is cleaner, no rubber caps are needed, the rolled tubes are more regular, and the gelatin does not touch the cotton plug, as is always the case in the tubes rolled under water, because of the impossibility of holding them steady at one level.

There is an impression that Esmarch tubes are not a success when made from ordinary nutrient agar-agar because of the tendency of this medium to collapse and fall into the bottom of the tube. This slipping down of the agar-agar is due to the water that is squeezed from it during solidification getting between the medium and the walls of the tube. This can easily be overcome by allowing the rolled tubes to remain at nearly a horizontal position, the cotton end of the tube about 1.5 to 2 cm. higher than the bottom of the tube, for twenty-four hours after rolling them. During this time the edge of the agar-agar nearest the cotton plug becomes dried and adherent to the walls of the tube, while the water collects at the most dependent point, *i.e.*, the bottom of the tube. After this they may be retained in the upright position without fear of the agar-agar slipping down. We have followed this process for several years with entire satisfaction.

In all these processes, if the dilutions of the number of organisms have been properly conducted, the results will be the same. The original plate or tube, as a rule, will be of no use because of the great number of colonies contained in it. Plate or tube No. 2 may be of service, but plate or tube 3 will usually contain the organisms in such small numbers that the colonies originating from them will have nothing to prevent their characteristic development.

For reasons of economy, the "original," tube 1, is sometimes substituted by a tube containing normal salt solution (0.6 to 0.7 per cent. of sodium chloride in water), which is thrown aside as soon as the dilutions are completed and only plates or tubes 2 and 3 are made.

CHAPTER IX.

The incubator used in bacteriological work—Gas-pressure regulator—Thermo-regulator—The form of burner employed in heating the incubator.

THE INCUBATOR.—When the plates have been made, it must be borne in mind that for the development of certain forms of bacteria a higher temperature is necessary than for the growth of others. The pathogenic or disease-producing organisms all grow more luxuriantly at the temperature of the human body (37.5° C.) than at lower temperatures; whereas, with the ordinary saprophytic forms almost any temperature between 18° to 20° C. and that of the body is favorable. It therefore becomes necessary to provide some place in which a constant temperature suitable to the growth of the pathogenic organisms can be maintained. For this purpose there have been devised a number of different forms of apparatus. Fundamentally they are all based upon the same principles, however, and a general description of the essential points involved in their construction will be all that is needed here.

This apparatus has the names thermostat, incubator, and brooding oven. It is a copper chamber (Fig. 16) with double walls, the space between which is filled with water. The incubating chamber may be opened or closed by a closely fitting double door, inside of which is usually a false door of glass through which the contents of the chambers may be inspected without actually opening it.

The whole apparatus is encased in either abestos boards or thick felt to prevent radiation of heat and consequent fluctuations in temperature. In the top of the chamber

Fig. 16.

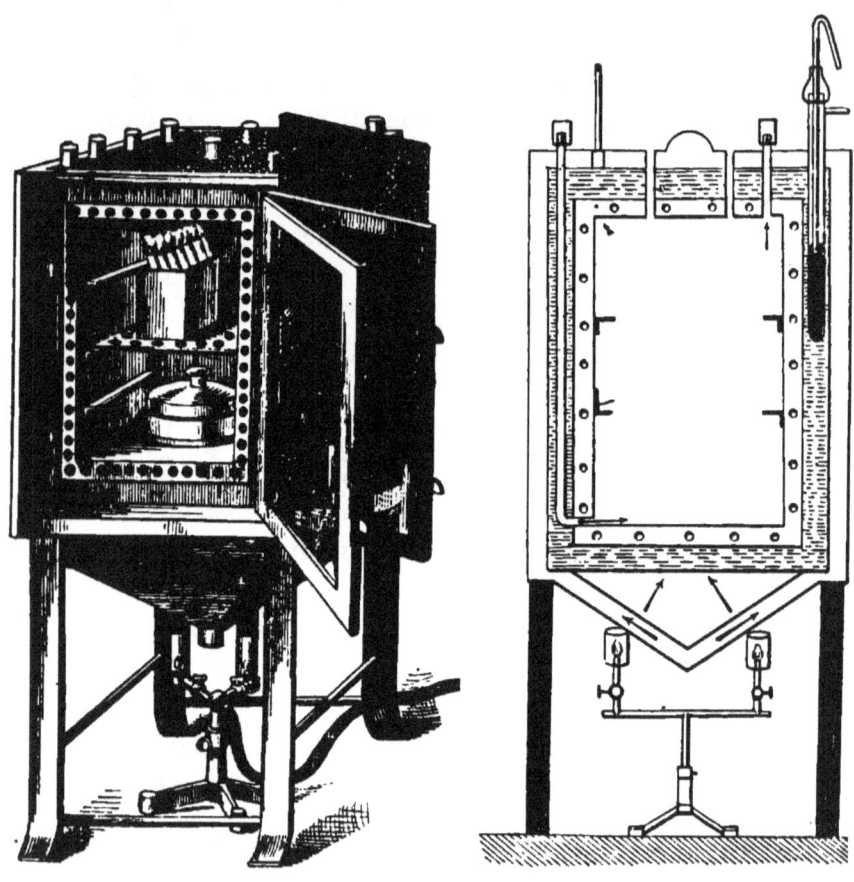

is a small opening through which a thermometer projects into its interior. At either corner, leading into the space containing the water are other openings, for the reception of another thermometer and a thermo-regulator, and for refilling the apparatus as the water evaporates.

On the side is a water-gauge for showing the level of the water between the walls. The object of the water chamber, which is formed by the double wall arrangement, is to insure by means of the warmed water an equable temperature at all parts of the apparatus—at the top as well as at the sides, back, and bottom. The apparatus should be kept filled with water, otherwise the object for which it is constructed will not be accomplished. When the chamber between the walls is filled with water the apparatus is heated from a gas-flame which is placed beneath it.

FIG. 17.

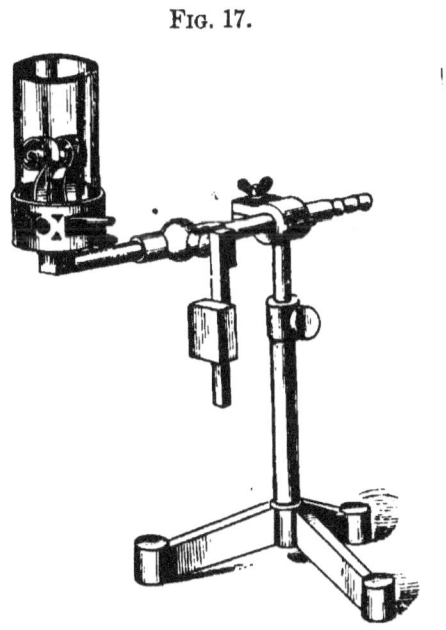

The burner employed in heating the incubator is known as "Koch's safety burner" (Fig. 17). It is a Bunsen burner provided with an arrangement for automatically turning off the gas supply and thus preventing accidents should the flame become extinguished at a time when no one was near. The gas-cock is provided with a long arm which is weighted and which, when the gas is turned on and burning, rests upon the end of a metal spiral which is heated by the flame. If by draughts or any other accident the flame becomes extinguished the metal spiral cools, and in cooling contracts and allows the weighted arm of the gas-cock to fall. By its falling the gas supply is turned off.

THERMO-REGULATORS.—The regulation and maintenance of the proper temperature within the incubator is accomplished by the employment of an automatic thermo-regulator.

The form of thermo-regulator used for this purpose is constructed upon principles involving the expansion and contraction of fluid substances under the influence of heat and cold. By means of this expansion and contraction, the amount of gas passing from the source of supply to the burner may be either diminished or increased as the temperature of the substance in which the regulator is placed either rises or falls.

The simplest form of thermo-regulator which serves to illustrate the principles involved is seen in Fig. 18.

It consists of a glass cylinder e, having a communicating branch tube b, and rubber stoopper f, through which projects the bent tube a. The tube a is ground to a slanting point at the extremity which projects into the tube e, and is provided a short distance above this point with a capillary opening g, in one of its sides.

When ready for use the cylinder e is filled with fluid, either mercury, calcium chloride solution, alcohol and ether, or a number of other substances depending upon the temperature to which it is to be subjected, up to about the level shown in the cut. It is then allowed to stand or is suspended in the bath the temperature of which it is to regulate. The rubber tubing coming from the gas supply is attached to the outer end of the glass tube a, and

Fig. 18.

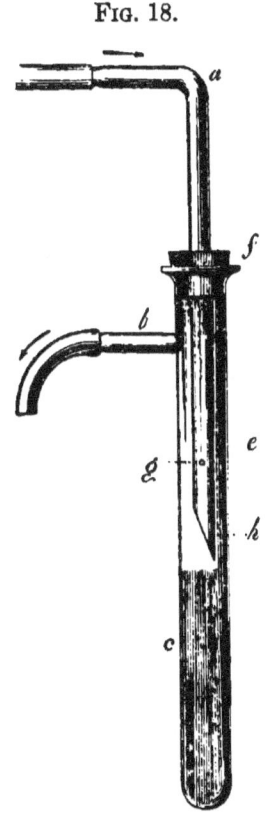

the tube going to the burner is slipped over the branch tube b. The gas is turned on and the burner lighted and placed under the bath. The gas now streams through the tube a into the cylinder e and out at b to the burner, but as the temperature of the bath rises, the fluid contained in the cylinder e, under the influence of the elevation of temperature begins to expand, and as a continuous rise in temperature proceeds, the expansion of the fluid accompanies it and gradually closes the slanting opening h of tube a. In this way the supply of gas becomes diminished and the rise in temperature of the bath will be less rapid, until finally the opening at h will be closed entirely, when the supply of gas to the burner will now be limited to that passing through the capillary opening g. This is not sufficient to maintain the highest temperature reached, and a gradual contraction of the fluid now occurs until there is again an outflow of gas from the opening h, when again the temperature rises. This contraction and expansion of the fluid in the regulator continues until eventually a point is reached at which the position of the fluid in the cylinder e allows of the passage of just enough gas from the opening h to maintain a constant temperature. This, in short, is the principle on which thermo-regulators are constructed, but it must be borne in mind that a great deal of detail exists in the construction of an accurate instrument. The number of different forms of this apparatus is comparatively large, and form has each its special merits.

The value, that is, the delicacy of the thermo-regulator depends upon a number of factors, all of which it would be useless to introduce into a book of this kind, but in general it may be said that the essential points to be observed in selecting a thermo-regulator depend in the main upon the temperatures to which it is to be applied. For low temperatures such fluids as ether, alcohol, and calcium chloride solution, which expand and contract rapidly and regularly under slight variations in temperature, are commonly employed; whereas for temperatures approaching the boiling-point of water mercury is most frequently used.

The temperature of the incubator is to be regulated, then, by the use of some such form of apparatus as that just described. It should be of sufficient delicacy to prevent a fluctuation of more than 0.2° C. in the temperature of the air within the chamber of the apparatus.

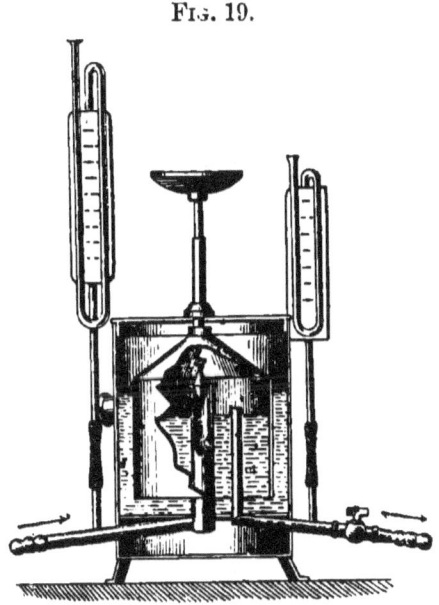

Fig. 19.

GAS-PRESSURE REGULATORS.—A gas-pressure regulator is not rarely intervened between the gas supply and the thermo-regulator. This apparatus has for its object the maintenance of a constant pressure of the gas going to the thermo-regulator. There are several instruments of this form in use, but none of them accomplishes the object for which they are designed.

The instrument most commonly employed, the apparatus of Moitessier (Fig. 19), is based on somewhat the same principles as the large regulators seen at the manufactories of illuminating gas, which act very well when employed on the large scale, as one sees them there; but which, when applied to the limited and sudden fluctuations seen in the gas coming from an ordinary gascock, are practically useless. They are too gross in their construction, and are only seen to act under comparatively great and gradual fluctuations in pressure. If a good form of thermo-regulator is employed, there is no necessity for the use of any of the forms of pressure-regulators thus far introduced.

CHAPTER X.

The study of colonies—Their naked-eye peculiarities and their appearance under different conditions—Differences in the structure of colonies from different species of bacteria—Stab cultures—Slant cultures.

THE plates upon agar-agar which have been prepared from a mixture of organisms and have been placed in the incubator, and those of gelatin which have been maintained at the ordinary temperature of the room, are usually ready for examination after twenty-four to forty-eight hours. They will be found to be marked here and there by small points or little islands of more or less opaque appearance. In some instances these will be so transparent that it is with difficulty one can see them with the naked eye. Again, they may be of a dense opaque appearance, at one time sharply circumscribed and round, again irregular in their outline. Here a point will present one color, there perhaps another. On gelatin some of the points will be seen to be lying on the surface of the medium, while others will be in the centre of a slight depression, the result of liquefaction of the gelatin about this point.

Place the plate containing these points upon the stage of the microscope and examine them with the lowest power objective, and again differences will be observed. Some of these minute points will be finely granular, others coarsely so; some will present a radiated appearance, while a neighbor may be concentrically arranged.

Here nothing particularly characteristic will present, there the point may resolve itself into a little mass having somewhat the appearance of a very small pellicle of raw cotton. All these differences, and many more, aid us in saying that these little points must be different in their nature. With a pointed platinum needle take up a bit of one of these little islands, prepare a stained cover-slip preparation (see chapter on cover-slip preparations) from it, and examine it under the high power oil-immersion objective, under access of the greatest amount of light afforded by the illuminator of the microscope. The preparation will be seen to be made up entirely of bodies of the same shape; they will all be spheres, or ovals, or rods, but not a mixture of these forms, if proper care in the manipulation has been taken. Examine in the same way a neighboring spot which possesses different naked-eye appearances, and it will be found to consist of bodies of an entirely different appearance from those in the first preparation.

These spots or islands on the surface of the plates are colonies of bacteria, differing severally; not only in outward appearances, the one from the other, but, as our cover-slip preparations show, in the morphological characteristics of the individual organisms composing them. If from one of these colonies a second set of plates be prepared, the peculiarities which were at first observed in this colony will be reproduced in the new set of colonies which develop. In other words, these peculiarities are constant under constant conditions. The colonies will be found to consist of the same organisms as the colony from which the plates were made, and colonies of no other organisms will be present.

With all organisms differences in the appearance of

the colonies depending upon their location in the medium can usually be detected. When deep down in the medium, owing to surrounding pressure, they are quite round, oval, or lozenge-shape; whereas, when they are on the surface of the gelatin or agar, they may take quite a different form. This is purely a mechanical effect, and is always to be borne in mind, otherwise errors are apt to arise.

PURE CULTURES.—If from one of these small colonies a bit be taken upon the point of a *sterilized* platinum needle and introduced into a tube of sterilized gelatin or agar-agar, the growth that results will be what is known as a "pure culture," the condition in which all organisms must be before a systematic study of their many pecularities is begun. Sometimes several series of plates are necessary before the organism can be obtained pure, but by patiently following this plan the results will ultimately be satisfactory.

TEST-TUBE CULTURES; STAB CULTURES; SMEAR CULTURES.—After separating the organisms, the one from the other by the plate method just described, they must be isolated from the plates as pure stab or smear cultures.

This is done in the following way: Decide upon the colony from which the pure culture is to be made. Select preferably a small colony and one as widely separated from other colonies as possible. Sterilize in the gas-flame a straight platinum-wire needle. The glass handle of the needle should be drawn through the flame as well as the needle itself, otherwise contamination from this source may occur. When it is cool, which is in three to five seconds, take up carefully a portion of the colony. Guard against touching *anything but the colony*. If, during manipulation, the needle touches *anything else whatever* than the colony from which the culture is to be made, it must be sterilized again. This holds not only for the time before touching the colony, but also during its passage into the test-tube from the colony, otherwise there is no guarantee that the growth resulting from the inoculation of this bit of colony into a fresh sterile medium will be pure.

In the meantime have in the other hand a test-tube of sterile medium : gelatin, agar-agar, or potato. This tube is held across the palm of the hand in an almost horizontal position with its mouth pointing out between the thumb and index finger and its contents toward the body of the worker. With the disengaged fingers of the hand holding the needle, the cotton plug is removed from the tube by a twisting motion and placed between the index and second fingers of the hand holding the tube in such a way that the portion of the plug which fits into the mouth of the test-tube looks toward the dorsal surface of the hand and *does not touch any portion of the hand*—this is accomplished by placing *only the overhanging* portion of the plug between the fingers. The needle containing the bit of colony is now to be thrust into the medium in the tube if a stab culture is desired, or rubbed gently over its surface if a smear culture is to be made. The needle is then withdrawn, the cotton plug replaced, *and the needle sterilized* before it is laid down. Neither the needle nor its handle should touch the inner sides of the test-tube if it can be avoided.

The tube is then labelled and set aside for observation. The growth which appears in the tube after twenty-four to thirty-six hours will be a pure culture of the organisms of which the colony was composed.

Cultures of this form are not only useful as a means of preserving pure cultures of the different organisms with which we may be working, but serve also to bring out certain characteristics of different organisms when grown in this way.

If gelatin is employed and the organism which has been introduced into it possesses the power of bringing about liquefaction, this result is by no means of the same appearance for all organisms. Some organisms cause a liquefaction which spreads across the whole upper surface of the gelatin and continues gradually downward; again it occurs in a funnel shape, the broad end of the funnel being uppermost and the point downward, corresponding to the track of the needle. At times a stocking- or sac-formed liquefaction may be noticed.

Obtain a number of organisms from different sources in pure cultures by the method given. Plant them as pure cultures, all at the same time, in gelatin—preferably gelatin of the same making—retain them under the same conditions of temperature, and note the finer differences in the way in which liquefaction occurs.

CHAPTER XI.

Systematic study of an organism—Steps necessary in identifying an organism as a definite species.

AFTER isolating an organism by the plate method, considerable work is necessary in order to establish its identity as a definite species.

It must possess certain morphological and cultural peculiarities, which must be constant under constant conditions.

Its form at certain stages must always be the same. Its ability or inability to produce spores must not vary under proper conditions. Its growth upon the different media under constant conditions of temperature must always present the same outward appearances. The reactions given by it to the media in which it is growing must follow a fixed rule. Its power to produce liquefaction of the gelatin, or to grow upon it without bringing about this change, must always be the same. Its motility or non-motility must be determined. Its production of certain chemical products must be detected by chemical analysis. Its behavior toward oxygen—*i. e.*, does it require this gas for its growth? is this gas an indifferent factor? or by its presence are the life processes of the organism checked?—must be determined. Its behavior under varying conditions of temperature and under the influence of different chemical bodies as well as its growth in media of different reactions are to be studied. The property of producing fermentation with the liberation of gases must be ascertained; and lastly, we must consider its behavior when introduced into the bodies of animals used for experimental work—*i. e.*, is it a disease-producing organism, or does it belong to the group of innocent saprophytes?

We have learned the methods for obtaining colonies, and have studied some of the peculiarities which are to distinguish them from one another. The next important step is to determine the morphology of the individuals composing these colonies as well as their relation to each other in the colony. These points are decided by microscopic examination of bits of the colony which have been transferred to thin glass cover-slips, upon which they are dried, stained, and mounted. Cover-slips for this purpose are prepared in two ways: either by taking up a bit of the colony on a needle, smearing it upon a cover-slip, staining it, and examining it—by which only the morphology of the individuals can be made out—or by the method of "impression cover-slip preparations," by which not only the morphology, but also the relation of the organisms to one another in the colony can be determined. The details of these methods will be found in the chapter on the methods of staining.

MICROSCOPIC EXAMINATION OF PREPARATIONS.

THE DIFFERENT PARTS OF THE MICROSCOPE.—Before describing the process of examining preparations microscopically, a few definitions of the terms used in referring to the microscope may not be out of place.

The ocular or *eye-piece* is the lens at which the eye is placed in looking through the instrument.

The objective is the lens which is at the distal end of

the barrel of the instrument, and which serves to magnify the object to be examined.

The stage is the shelf or platform of the microscope on which the object rests.

The reflector is the mirror placed beneath the stage, which serves to direct the light to the object to be examined.

The coarse adjustment is the rack-and-pinion arrangement by which the barrel of the microscope can be quickly raised or lowered.

The fine adjustment serves to raise and lower the barrel of the instrument very slowly and gradually.

For the microscopic study of bacteria it is essential that the microscope be provided with an oil-immersion system and a sub-stage condensing apparatus.

The Oil-immersion System consists in an objective so constructed that it can only be used when the media through which the light passes in entering it are all of the same index of refraction—*i. e.*, are homogeneous. This is accomplished by interposing between the face of the lens and the cover-slip covering the object to be examined a body which refracts the light in the same way as do the glass slide, the cover-slip, and the glass of which the objective is made. For this purpose a drop of oil of the same index of refraction as the glass is placed upon the face of the lens, and the examinations are made through this oil. There is thus no loss of light from deflection, as is the case in the dry systems.

The sub-stage condensing apparatus is a system of lenses situated beneath the central opening of the stage. They serve to condense the light passing from the reflector to the object in such a way that it is focussed upon the object. Between the condenser and reflector is placed an adjustable diaphragm, the aperture of which can be regulated, as circumstances require, to permit of either a very small or very large amount of light passing to the object.

MICROSCOPIC EXAMINATION OF COVER-SLIPS.—The stained cover-slip is to be examined with the oil-immersion objective, and with the diaphragm of the sub-stage condensing apparatus open to its full extent. The object gained by allowing the light to enter in such a large volume is that the contrast produced by the colored bacteria in the brightly illuminated field is much more conspicuous than when a smaller amount of light is thrown upon them. This is true not only for bacteria on cover-slips, but likewise for their differentiation from surrounding objects when they are located in tissues. With unstained bacteria and tissues, on the contrary, the structure can best be made out by reducing the bundle of light-rays to its smallest amount, and in this way favoring, *not color contrast*, but contrasts which appear as lights and shadows due to the differences in permeability to light of the various parts of the material under examination.

STEPS IN EXAMINING STAINED PREPARATIONS WITH THE OIL-IMMERSION SYSTEM.—Place upon the centre of the cover-slip which covers the preparation a small drop of immersion oil. Place the slide upon the centre of the stage of the microscope. With the coarse adjustment lower the oil-immersion objective until it *just touches* the drop of oil. Open the illuminating apparatus to its full extent. Then, with the eye to the microscope and the hand on the fine adjustment, turn the adjusting-screw toward *the right* until the field becomes somewhat colored in appearance. When this is seen, proceed more slowly in the same direction, and, after one or two turns, the object will be in focus. *Do not remove the eye from the instrument until this has been accomplished.*

Then, with one hand upon the fine adjustment and the thumb and index finger of the other hand holding lightly the slide by its end, the slide may be moved about under the objective. At the same time the screw of the fine adjustment must be turned back and forth so that the different levels of the preparation may one after the other be brought into focus. In this way the whole section or preparation may be inspected. When the examination is finished, raise the objective from the preparation by turning the screw of the *coarse* adjustment *toward you*. Remove the preparation from the stage, and, with a fine silk cloth or handkerchief, *wipe very gently and carefully* the oil from the face of the lens. The lens is then unscrewed from the microscope and placed in the case intended for its reception.

During work, of course, the lens need not be cleaned and put away after each examination; but when the work for the day is over, an immersion lens must always be protected in this way. Under no circumstances should it be allowed to remain in the immersion oil or exposed to dust for any length of time.

EXAMINATION OF UNSTAINED PREPARATIONS.— "*Hanging drops.*" It frequently becomes necessary to examine bacteria in the unstained condition. The circumstances calling for this arise while studying the multiplication of cells, the germination of spores, the formation of spores, and the absence or presence of motility.

In this method the organisms to be studied are suspended in a drop of salt solution or bouillon in the

MICROSCOPIC EXAMINATIONS. 109

centre of a cover-slip. This is then placed, drop down, upon an object-glass in the centre of which a hollow or depression is ground (Fig. 20). The slip is held in position by a thin layer of vaselin, which may be painted

FIG. 20.

around the margins of the depression. This not only prevents the slip from moving from its position during examination, but also prevents drying by evaporation if the preparation is to be observed for any length of time. This is known as the "hanging drop" method of examination or cultivation. It is indispensable for the purposes mentioned, and at the same time requires considerable care in its manipulation. The fluid is so transparent that the cover-slip is often broken and the face of the objective injured by its being brought down upon the preparation before one is aware that the focal distance has been reached. This may be avoided by grasping the slide with the left hand and moving it back and forth under the objective as it is brought down toward the object. As soon as the *least pressure* is felt upon the slide the objective must be raised, otherwise the cover-slip will be broken and the lens may be rendered worthless.

A safer plan is to bring the edge of the drop into the centre of the field with one of the higher power dry lenses. When this is accomplished, substitute the immersion for the dry system, and the edge of the drop can now easily be found.

In examining bacteria by this method there is a possibility of error that must be guarded against. All microscopic insoluble particles in suspension in fluids possess a peculiar tremor or vibratory motion, the so-called "Brownian motion." This is very apt to give the impression that the organisms under examination are motile when in truth they are not so, their movement in the fluid being due only to this molecular tremor.

The difference between the motion of bodies which are undergoing this molecular tremor and that possessed by certain living bacteria is that the former particles never move from their place in the field, while the living bacteria alter their position in relation to the surrounding organisms, and may dart from one position in the field to another. With some cases the true movement of bacteria is very slow and undulating, while in others it is rapid and darting. The molecular tremor may be seen with non-motile and with dead organisms.

Prepare three hanging-drop preparations, one from a drop of dilute India ink, a second from a culture of micrococci, and a third from a culture of the bacillus of typhoid fever. In what way do they differ?

STUDY OF SPORE-FORMATION.—The hanging-drop method just mentioned is not only employed for the detection of the motility of an organism, but for the study of its spore-forming properties.

Since with aërobic organisms spore-formation occurs, as a rule, only in the presence of oxygen, and is induced more by limitation of the nutrition of the organisms than by any other factor, it is essential that these two points should be borne in mind in preparing the drop cultures in which the process is to be studied. For this reason the drop of bouillon should be small and the air-chamber relatively large.

The cover-slip and hollow-ground slide should be carefully sterilized, and with a sterilized platinum loop a very small drop of bouillon is placed in the centre of the cover-slip. The slip is then inverted over the hollow depression in the sterilized object-glass and sealed with vaselin. The most convenient method of performing this last step in the process is to paint a ring of vaselin around the edges of the hollow in the slide, and then, without taking the cover-slip up from the table upon which it rests, invert the hollow over the drop and press it gently down upon the cover-slip. The vaselin causes the slip to adhere to the slide, so that it can be easily taken up. The drop now hangs in the centre of the small air-tight chamber which exists between the depression in the slide and the cover-slip. (See Fig. 20.)

A drop of sterilized agar-agar may be substituted for the bouillon. It serves to retain the organisms in a fixed position, and the process may be more easily followed.

As soon as finished, the preparation is to be examined microscopically, and the condition of the organisms noted. It is then to be retained in a warm chamber especially devised for the purpose and kept under continuous observation. The form of chamber best adapted for the purpose is one which envelops the whole microscope. It is provided with a window through which the light enters, and an arrangement for moving the slide about from the outside. The formation of spores requires a much longer time than the germination of spores into bacilli, but with patience both processes may be satisfactorily observed.

It will be noticed that the description of this process

is very much like that which has just been given, but differs from it in one respect, viz., that in this manipulation we are not making a preparation which is simply to be examined and then thrown aside, but it is an actual pure culture, and must be kept as such, otherwise the observation will be worthless. For this reason the greatest care must be observed in the sterilization of all objects employed. Studies upon spore-formation by this method frequently continue over hours, and sometimes days, and contamination must, therefore, be carefully guarded against. The study should be begun with the vegetative form of the organism; the hanging-drop preparation should, for this reason, always be made from a perfectly fresh culture of the organism under consideration, before time has elapsed for spores to form.

The simple detection of the presence or absence of spore-formation can in many cases be made by other methods. For example, many species of bacteria which possess this property form spores most readily upon media from which it is somewhat difficult for them to obtain the necessary nutrition; potatoes and agar-agar which have become a little dry offer very favorable conditions, because of the limited area from which the growing bacteria can draw their nutritive supplies and because of the free access which they have to oxygen; for, their growth being on the surface, they are surrounded by this gas unless means are taken to prevent it. By the hanging-drop method, however, more than this simple property may be determined. It is possible not only to detect the stages and steps in the formation of endogenous spores, but when the spores are completely formed by transferring them to a fresh bouillon-drop or drop of agar-agar, preserved in the same way, their germination into mature rods may be seen. The word rods is used because as yet we have no evidence that endogenous spore-formation occurs in any of the other morphological groups of bacteria.

STUDY OF GELATIN CULTURES.—As has been previously stated, the behavior of bacteria toward gelatin differs—some of them producing apparently no alteration in the medium, while others bring about a form of peptonization which results in liquefaction of the gelatin at and around the place at which the colonies are growing. In some instances this liquefaction spreads laterally, in others it sinks directly down into the gelatin. These differences have been conspicuously shown and employed as one of the means of differentiation of otherwise closely allied members of the same family of bacteria. Studies upon the organism of Asiatic cholera and a number of closely allied forms reveal a decided difference in the manner of liquefaction produced by these different organisms. The slightest detail in this respect must be noted, and its frequency or constancy under different conditions determined.

CULTURES ON POTATO.—A very important feature in the study of an organism is its growth on sterilized potato. Many organisms present appearances under this method of cultivation which alone can almost be considered characteristic. In some cases coarsely lobulated, elevated, dry or moist patches of development occur after a few hours; again, the growth may be finely granular and but slightly elevated above the surface of the potato; at one time it will be dry and dull in appearance, again it may be moist and glistening. Sometimes there is a production of bubbles, owing to fermentation brought about by the growth of the organs.

A most striking form of development on potato is that possessed by the organism of typhoid fever and the bacillus of diphtheria. After the inoculation of a potato with either of these organisms there is no naked-eye evidence of a growth in either instance, though microscopic examination of scrapings from the surface of the potato reveals an active multiplication of the organisms which had been planted there. The potato is one of the most important differential media which we possess for this work.

REACTION PRODUCED BY ORGANISMS IN THEIR GROWTH.—The reactions produced in the media by different organisms in the course of their growth are very valuable as means of differentiation.

In some cases these changes are so marked that they are readily detected by the coarser reagents; again they are so slight as to require the employment of the most delicate indicators. They are sometimes seen to produce at one period of their growth an alkaline, at another period an acid reaction. This is seen in the cultures of the bacillus diphtheriæ of Löffler.

These differences are best seen after the addition to the media in which the organisms are to grow of some of the chemical substances which do not interfere with the development of the organisms, but which under one reaction are of one color, and with an alteration of the reaction become a different color, the change being indicated by the play of colors. Such substances as litmus, in the form of tincture, and coralline (rosolic acid) in alcoholic solution have been employed for this purpose. They may be added to the media in the proportions given in the chapter on media, and the alterations in their colors studied with different bacteria.

Milk and litmus tincture or peptone solution to which rosolic acid has been added are very favorable media for this experiment.

In milk, coagula will now and then appear as a result of acids produced during the bacterial life, while again acids may be produced and yet no coagulation be noticed.

ANILINE DYES FOR DIFFERENTIAL DIAGNOSIS.— The addition to solid media of some of the aniline dyes, fuchsin, methylene-blue, methylene-green, and several others, as well as combinations of these dyes, have been recommended as a means of differentiation of organisms, the differences consisting in alterations in the color of the media due to oxidizing or reducing properties of the growing bacteria. As yet but little has come from this method of work. It cannot at present be recommended as a reliable means of diagnosis.

BEHAVIOR TOWARD STAINING REAGENTS.—The behavior of certain organisms toward the different dyes and their reactions under special methods of after-treatment serve as aids to their diagnosis. With very few exceptions all bacteria stain readily with the common aniline dyes, but they differ materially in the tenacity with which they retain these colors under the subsequent treatment with decolorizing agents.

The tubercle bacillus and the bacillus of leprosy, for example, are difficult to stain, but when once stained retain their color under the action of such energetic decolorizing agents as alcohol, nitric acid, oxalic acid, etc.

Certain other organisms when stained with a solution of gentian violet in aniline-water, retain their color when treated with such decolorizing bodies as iodine solution and alcohol (Gram's method), while again others are completely decolorized by this method.

Many of them can only be treated with water, or but for a few seconds with alcohol, without losing their color.

It is essential that these peculiarities should be carefully noted in studying an organism.

FERMENTATION.—The production of gas as an indication of fermentation is an accompaniment of the growth of some organisms. This is best studied in media to which 1 to 2 per cent. of grape sugar has been added.

In this experiment the test-tube should be filled to about one-half its volume with agar-agar. The medium is then liquefied, and when at the proper temperature, a small quantity of a pure culture of the organism under consideration should be carefully distributed through it. The tube is then placed into icewater and rapidly solidified in the vertical position. When solid it is placed in the incubator. After twenty-four to thirty-six hours, if the organism possesses the property of causing fermentation of sugar, the medium will be dotted everywhere with very small cavities containing the gas that has resulted.

Where it is important that the nature of the gas thus produced should be studied, it must be collected, and a special form of apparatus is employed. The cultivation is now to be conducted in a fluid medium. The fermentation flasks of somewhat the pattern of that used by Einhorn in the fermentation test for sugar in the urine serve very well for this purpose.

CULTIVATION WITHOUT OXYGEN.—As we have already learned, there is a group of organisms to which the name "anaërobic organisms" has been given, which are characterized by their inability to grow in the presence of oxygen. For the cultivation of the members of this group a number of devices are employed for the exclusion of oxygen from the cultures.

Koch's method. Koch covered the surface of a gelatin plate, which had been previously inoculated, with a thin sheet of sterilized isinglass. The organisms which grew beneath it were supposed to grow without oxygen.

Hesse's method. Hesse poured sterilized oil upon the surface of a culture made by stabbing into a tube of gelatin. The growth that occurred along the track of the needle was supposed to be anaërobic in nature.

Method of Buchner. The plan suggested by Buchner of allowing the cultures to develop in an atmosphere robbed of its oxygen by pyrogallic acid gives very good results. In this method the culture, which is either a slant or stab culture in a test-tube, is placed—tube, cotton plug, and all—into a larger tube in the bottom of which has been deposited 1 gramme of pyrogallic acid and 10 c.c. of $\frac{1}{10}$ normal[1] caustic potash solution. The larger tube is then tightly plugged with a rubber

---

[1] A normal solution is one that contains in a litre as many grammmes of the dissolved substance as are indicated by its molecular equivalent. The equivalent is that amount of a chemical compound which possesses the same chemical value as does one atom of hydrogen. For example: One molecule of hydrochloric acid (HCl) has a molecular weight and also an equivalent weight of 36.5; a molecule of this acid has the same chemical value as one atom of hydrogen. Its normal solution is therefore 36.5 grammes to the litre. On the other hand, sulphuric acid (H_2SO_4) contains in each molecule two replaceable hydrogen atoms; its normal solution is not, therefore, 80 grammes (its molecular weight) to the litre, but that amount which would be equivalent chemically to one hydrogen atom, viz., 40 grammes (one-half its molecular weight) to the litre. A normal solution of caustic potash contains as many grammes to the litre as the number of its molecular weight—56.1 grammes to the litre of water.

stopper. The oxygen is quickly absorbed by the pyrogallic acid, and the organisms develop in the remaining constituents of the atmosphere—nitrogen, a small amount of CO_2, and a trace of ammonia.

Method of C. Fränkel. Carl Fränkel suggests the following method: The tube is first prepared as if for an ordinary Esmarch tube. The cotton plug is then replaced by a rubber stopper, through which pass two glass tubes. These have all been sterilized in the steam sterilizer before using. On the outer side of the stopper these two tubes are bent at right angles to the long axis of the test-tube into which they are to be placed, and both are slightly drawn out in the gas flame. At the outer extremity of both of these tubes a plug of cotton is placed; this is to prevent access of foreign organisms during manipulation. At the inner side of the rubber stopper—that is, the end which is to be inserted into the test-tube—the glass tubes are of different lengths: one reaches to within 0.5 cm. of the bottom of the test-tube, the other is cut off flush with the under surface of the stopper. This rubber stopper, with its glass tubes, is to replace the cotton plug of the test-tube; the outer end of the longer glass tube is then connected with a hydrogen generator and hydrogen is allowed to bubble through the gelatin in the tube until all contained air has been expelled and its place taken by the hydrogen. The organisms are to grow, then, in an atmosphere of hydrogen. When all air has been expelled, the two external ends of the glass tubes are to be sealed in the gas-flame at the portions where they have been drawn out. In sealing the tubes in the gas-flame one must be sure that all air has been expelled, otherwise an explosion is inevitable. This may be accomplished by allowing the hydrogen to bubble through the gelatin for about ten minutes. The rubber stopper is then painted around with melted paraffin and the tube rolled in the way given for ordinary Esmarch tubes.

During the operation the tube containing the liquefied gelatin should be kept in a water-bath of a temperature which will prevent its solidifying and at the same time not kill the organisms with which it has been inoculated.

Method of Liborius. Another method, that of Liborius, is to fill a test-tube about three-quarters full of gelatin. This is kept at the temperature of boiling water for ten minutes to expel all air from it. It is then to be rapidly cooled in ice-water, and, when between 30° C. and 40° C., is to be inoculated, and the gelatin rapidly solidified. It is then to be sealed up in the flame.

Method of Kitasato and Weil. For favoring the anaërobic conditions, Kitasato and Weil have suggested the addition to the culture media of some strong reducing agent. They recommend formic acid in 0.3 to 0.5 per cent.

Esmarch's method. Esmarch's plan is to prepare in the usual way an Esmarch tube of the organisms, and this is to be subjected to a low temperature, and while quite cold is filled with liquefied gelatin, and the whole allowed to solidify rapidly. In this method the colonies develop along the sides of the tubes, and can more easily be studied than where they are mixed through the gelatin, as in the method of Liborius.

By some workers the oxygen is removed by actual pumping with the air-pump.

Many other methods exist for this special purpose, but for the beginner those given will suffice.

INDOL PRODUCTION.—The production of products other than those which give rise to alterations in the reaction of the media, and whose presence may be detected by simple chemical reactions, is now a recognized step in the identification of different species of bacteria. Among these chemical products there is one which is produced by a number of organisms, and whose presence may easily be detected by its characteristic behavior when treated with certain substances.

Indol, when acted upon by reducing agents, is seen to become of a more or less conspicuous rose color. This body was recognized some time ago as one of the products of growth of the comma bacillus of Asiatic cholera, and for a time was thought to characterize the changes produced in the media through the growth of this organism. It has since been found that there exist other bacteria which also possess the property of producing this body in the course of their development.

The method employed for its detection is as follows: Cultivate the organism for twenty-four to forty-eight hours at a temperature of 37° C., in the simple peptone solution known as "Dunham's solution" (see formula for this medium). This solution is preferred because its pale color does not mask the rose color of the reaction when the amount of indol present is very small.

Four tubes should always be inoculated and kept under exactly the same conditions for the same length of time.

At the end of twenty-four or forty-eight hours the test may be made. Proceed as follows: To a tube containing 7 c.c. of the peptone solution, but which has *not* been inoculated, add 10 drops of concentrated sulphuric acid. To another similar tube add 1 c.c. of a 0.01 per cent. solution of sodium nitrite, and afterward 10 drops of concentrated sulphuric acid. Observe the tubes for five to ten minutes. No alteration in their color appears, or at least there will be no production of a rose color. They contain no indol.

Treat in the same way, with the acid alone, two of the tubes which *have been inoculated.* If no rose color appears after five or ten minutes, add 1 c.c. of the sodium nitrite solution. If now no rose color is produced, the indol reaction may be considered as negative. No indol is present.

If indol is present, and the rose color appears after the addition of the acid alone, it is plain that not only indol has been formed, but likewise a reducing body. This is found, by proper means, to be nitrous acid. The sulphuric acid liberates it from its salts and permits of its reducing action being seen.

If the rose color appears only after the addition of both the acid and the nitrite solution, then indol has been formed during the growth of the organisms, but no nitrites.

Control the results obtained by treating the two remaining cultures in the same way.

CHAPTER XII.

Methods of staining—Solutions employed—Preparation and staining of cover-slips—Preparation of tissues for section-cutting—Staining of tissues—Special staining methods.

THE entire list of solutions and methods which have been recommended for the staining of bacteria are not essential to the work of the beginner, so that only those methods which are of most common application will be given in this book. In general, it suffices to say, bacteria stain best with watery solutions of the basic aniline dyes, and of these, fuchsin, gentian-violet, and methylene-blue are those most frequently employed.

In practical work bacteria require to be stained in two conditions: either dried upon cover-slips and then stained, or stained in sections of tissues in which they have been deposited during the course of disease. In both processes the essential point to be borne in mind is that the bacteria, because of their microscopic dimensions, require to be more conspicuously stained than the surrounding materials upon the cover-slips or in the sections, otherwise their differentiation is a matter of the greatest difficulty, if not of impossibility. For this reason, especially in the case of section staining, it frequently becomes necessary to decolorize the tissues after removing them from the staining solutions in order to render the bacteria more prominent; and for this purpose special methods, which provide for decolorization of the tissues without robbing the bacteria of their color, are employed. The ordinary method of cover-slip examination of bacteria, which is constantly in use in these studies, is performed in the following way:

COVER-SLIP PREPARATIONS.—In order that the distribution of the organisms upon the cover-slips may be uniform and in as thin a layer as possible, it is essential that the slip should be clean and free from grease. For cleansing the slips several methods may be employed.

The simplest plan with new cover-slips is to immerse them for a few hours in strong nitric acid, after which they are rinsed in water, then in alcohol, ether, and, finally, they may be kept in alcohol to which a little ammonia has been added. When they are to be used they should be wiped dry with a clean cotton or silk handkerchief.

If the slips have been previously used, boiling in strong soap solution, followed by rinsing in clean warm water, then treated as above, renders them clean enough for ordinary purposes.

A method commonly employed is to remove all coarse adherent matter from slips and slides by allowing them to remain for a time in strong nitric or sulphuric acid. They are removed from the acid after several days, rinsed off in water, and treated as above. Knauer has recently suggested the boiling of soiled cover-slips and slides for from twenty to thirty minutes in a 10 per cent. watery solution of lysol, after which they are to be carefully rinsed in water until all trace of the lysol has disappeared. They are then to be wiped dry with a clean handkerchief.

Löffler's method, which provides for the complete removal of all grease, is to warm the cover-slips in concentrated sulphuric acid for a time, then rinse them in water, after which they are kept in a mixture of equal parts of alcohol and ammonia. They are to be dried on a cloth from which the fat has been extracted.

Steps in making the preparations. Place upon the centre of one of the clean, dry cover-slips a very small drop of distilled water or physiological salt solution. With a platinum needle, which has been sterilized in the gas-flame *just before using* and allowed to cool, take up a very small portion of the colony to be examined and mix it carefully with the drop on the slip until there exists a very thin homogeneous film over the larger part of the surface. This is to be dried upon the slip by either allowing it to remain upon the table in the horizontal position under a cover, to protect it from dust, or by holding it *between the fingers (not with the forceps)*, at some distance above the gas-flame until it is quite dry. If held with the forceps over the flame at this stage, too much heat may be unconsciously applied, and the morphology of the organisms in the preparation distorted. When held between the fingers with the layer of bacteria *away from the flame* no such accident is likely to occur. When the whole pellicle is completely dried the slip is to be taken up with the forceps, and, holding the side upon which the bacteria are deposited away from the direct action of the flame, is to be passed through the flame three times, a little more than one second being allowed for each transit. Unless the preliminary drying at the low temperature has been complete, the preparation will be rendered worthless by the subsequent "fixing" at the higher temperature, for the reason that the protoplasm of bacteria when moist coagulates at these temperatures, and in doing so the normal outline of the cells is altered. If carefully dried before fixing, this does not occur and the morphology of the organism remains unchanged. A better plan for the process of fixing is to employ a copper plate of about 35 cm. long by 10 cm. wide by 0.3 cm. thick. This plate is laid upon an iron tripod and a small gas-flame is placed beneath one of its extremities. By this arrangement one can get a graduated temperature, beginning at the point of the plate above the gas-flame where it is hottest, and becoming gradually cooler toward the other end of the plate, which may be of a very low temperature. By dropping water upon the plate, beginning at the hottest point and proceeding toward the cooler end, it is easy to determine the point at which the water just boils; it is at a little below this point that the cover-slips are to be placed, bacteria side up, and allowed to remain about ten minutes, when the fixing will be complete. The same may be accomplished in a small copper drying-oven, which is regulated to remain at the temperature of 95° to 98° C. This plan is to be preferred to the process of passing the cover-slips through the flame, as the organisms are always subjected to the same degree of heat, and the distortions which sometimes occur from the too great and irregular application of high temperatures may in part be eliminated. The fixing consists in drying or coagulating the gelatinous envelope surrounding the organisms, by which means they are caused to adhere to the surface of the cover-slip. When fixed, the staining is usually a simple matter. The majority of bacteria with which the beginner will have to deal stain readily with solutions of any of the basic aniline dyes.

To stain the fixed preparation it is taken between the forceps, and a few drops of a watery solution of fuchsin, gentian-violet, or methylene-blue are placed upon the film and are allowed to remain there twenty to thirty seconds. The slip is then carefully rinsed in water, and without drying is placed *bacteria down* upon a slide, the excess of water is taken up with blotting-paper, and the preparation is ready for examination.

Another plan that is sometimes used is to bring the slip upon the slide, *bacteria down*, without rinsing off the staining fluid; the excess of fluid is removed with blotting-paper and the preparation is ready for examination with the microscope. This method is satisfactory and time-saving, but must always be practised with care. The staining fluid should always be carefully filtered before using, to rid it of insoluble particles which might mislead the examiner into mistaking them for bacteria. If upon examination the preparation proves to be of particular interest, so that it is desirable to preserve it, then it is to be mounted permanently. The drop of immersion oil is to be removed from the surface of the slip with blotting-paper, and the slip loosened from the slide by allowing water to flow around its edges. It is then taken up with the forceps, carefully deprived of the water adhering to it by means of blotting-paper, and then allowed to dry. When dry it is mounted in xylol-Canada balsam by placing a small drop of the balsam upon the surface of the film, and then inverting the slip upon a clean glass slide.

IMPRESSION COVER-SLIP PREPARATIONS.—The impression preparations differ in value from the ordinary cover-slip preparations only in one respect: they present an impression of the organisms as they were arranged in the colony from which the preparation was made. They are made by gently covering the colony with a thin, clean cover-slip, lightly pressing upon it, and, without moving the slip laterally, lifting it up by one of its edges. The organisms adhere to the slip in the same relation to one another that they had in the colony. The subsequent steps of drying, fixing, staining, and mounting are the same as those just given for the ordinary cover-slip preparations.

By this method, constancies in the arrangement and grouping of the individuals in a colony can often be made out. Some will always appear irregularly massed together, others will grow in parallel bundles, while others, again, will be seen as long twisted threads.

THE ORDINARY STAINING SOLUTIONS.—The solutions commonly employed in staining cover-slip preparations are, as has been stated, watery solutions of the basic aniline dyes — fuchsin, gentian-violet, and methylene-blue. These solutions may be prepared either by directly dissolving the dyes in substance in water until the proper degree of concentration has been reached, or by preparing them from concentrated watery or alcoholic solutions of the dyes which may be kept on hand as stock. The latter method is that commonly practised.

The solutions of the colors which are in constant use in staining are prepared as follows :

Prepare as stock, saturated alcoholic or watery solutions of fuchsin, gentian-violet, and methylene-blue. These solutions are best prepared by pouring into clean bottles, enough of the dyes in substance to fill them to about one-fourth their capacity. The bottle should then be filled with alcohol or with water, tightly corked, well shaken, and allowed to stand for twenty-four hours. If at the end of this time all the staining material has been dissolved, more should be added, the bottle being again shaken, and allowed to stand for another twenty-four hours; this must be repeated until a permanent sediment of undissolved coloring matter is seen upon the bottom of the bottle. This will then be labelled saturated alcoholic or watery solution of fuchsin, gentian-violet, or methylene-blue, as the case may be. *The alcoholic solutions will not answer for staining purposes.*

The solutions with which the staining is accomplished are made from these alcoholic solutions in the following way :

An ordinary test-tube of about 13 mm. diameter is three-fourths filled with distilled water and the concentrated alcoholic or watery solution of the dye is then

FIG. 21.

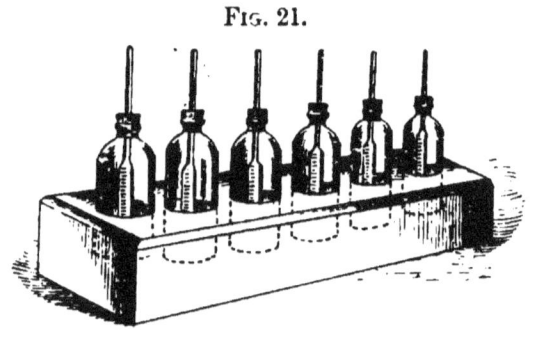

added, little by little, until one can just see through the solution. It is then ready for use. Care must be given that the color does not become too dense. The best results are obtained when it is *just transparent* as viewed through a layer of about 12 to 14 mm. thick.

These represent the staining solutions in everyday use. They are kept in bottles supplied with stoppers and pipettes (Fig. 21), and when used are dropped upon the preparation to be stained. After remaining upon the preparation for about thirty seconds, they are washed off in water and the preparation can then be examined.

For certain bacteria which stain only imperfectly with these simple solutions it is necessary to employ some agent that will increase the penetrating action of the dyes. Experience has taught us that this can be accomplished by the addition to the solutions of small quantities of alkaline substances or by dissolving the staining materials in strong watery solutions of either aniline oil or carbolic acid, instead of simple water.

Of the solutions thus prepared which may always be employed upon bacteria which show a tendency to stain imperfectly, there are three in common use—Löffler's alkaline methylene-blue solution, the Koch-Ehrlich aniline-water solution of either fuchsin, gentian-violet, or methylene-blue, and Ziehl's solution of fuchsin in carbolic acid. These solutions are as follows:

Löffler's alkaline methylene-blue solution:

Concentrated alcoholic solution of methylene-blue 30 c.c.
Caustic potash in 1 : 10,000 solution . . 100 c.c.

Koch-Ehrlich aniline-water solutions. To about 100 c.c. of distilled water aniline oil is added, drop by drop, and the solution thoroughly shaken after each addition until it is of an opaque appearance. It is then filtered through moistened filter-paper until the filtrate is perfectly clear. To 100 c.c. of the clear filtrate add 10 c.c. of absolute alcohol and 11 c.c. of the concentrated alcoholic solution of either fuchsin, methylene-blue, or gentian-violet, preferably fuchsin or gentian-violet.

Ziehl's carbolic-fuchsin solution:

Distilled water	100 c.c.
Carbolic acid (crystalline) . . .	5 grammes.
Alcohol	10 c.c.
Fuchsin in substance	1 gramme.

Or it may be prepared by adding to a 5 per cent. watery solution of carbolic acid the saturated alcoholic solution of fuchsin until a metallic lustre appears on the surface of the fluid.

Both the Koch-Ehrlich and the Ziehl solutions decompose very quickly after having been made, so that it is better to prepare them when needed in small quantities than to employ old solutions. Solutions older than seven to nine days should not be used.

The three solutions just given may be used for cover-glass preparations in the ordinary way.

In some manipulations it becomes necessary to stain the bacteria very intensely, so that they may retain their color when exposed to the action of decolorizing agents. These are usually employed for the purpose of depriving surrounding objects or tissues of their color in order that the stained bacteria may stand out in greater contrast. It is in these cases that the staining solution with which the bacteria are being treated is to be warmed, and in some cases boiled, so as to further increase its penetrating action. When so treated, certain of the bacteria will retain their color, even when exposed to very strong decolorizers. The tubercle bacillus is characterized from all other bacteria, except the bacillus of leprosy, by the tenacity with which it retains its color when treated in this way. It is an organism that is difficult to stain, but when once stained is equally difficult to rob of its color.

METHOD OF STAINING THE TUBERCLE BACILLUS.— Select from the sputum of a tuberculous subject one of the small, white, cheesy masses which it is seen to contain. Spread this upon a cover-slip and dry and fix it in the usual way. The slip is now to be taken by its edge with the forceps and the film covered with a few drops of either the solution of Koch-Ehrlich or of Ziehl. It is then held over the gas-flame, at first some distance away, gradually being brought nearer, until the fluid begins to boil. After it has bubbled up once or twice it is removed from the flame, the excess of staining washed away in a stream of water, and it is then immersed in a 30 per cent. solution of nitric acid in water and allowed to remain there until all the color has disappeared. In some cases this takes longer than in others. One can always determine if decolorization is complete by washing off the acid in a stream of water. If the preparation is still quite colored it should be again immersed in the acid; if of only a very faint color it may be dipped in alcohol, again washed off in water, and may now be stained with some contrast color. If, for example, the tubercle bacilli have been stained with fuchsin, methylene-blue forms a good contrast stain. In making the contrast stain the steps in the process are exactly those followed in the ordinary staining of cover-slip preparations in general: the slip containing the stained tubercle bacilli is rinsed off carefully in water and a few drops of the methylene-blue solution are placed upon it and allowed to remain for thirty to forty seconds, when it is again rinsed in water and examined microscopically. For the purpose of observing the difference between the behavior of the tubercle bacilli and the other organisms present in the preparation toward this method of staining, it is well to examine the preparation microscopically before the contrast stain is made, then remove it, give it the contrast color, and examine it again. It will be seen that before the contrast color has been given to the preparation the tubercle bacilli will be the only stained objects to be made out, and the preparation will appear devoid of other organisms, but upon examining it after it has received the contrast color, a great many other organisms will now appear; these will take on the second color employed, while the tubercle bacilli will retain their original color. Before decolorization all organisms in the preparation were of the same color, but during the application of the decolorizing solution all except the tubercle bacilli gave up their color. This characteristic, as said, serves to differentiate the tubercle bacillus from all other organisms, except the bacillus of leprosy, which stains in the same way as does the bacillus of tuberculosis. A number of different methods have been suggested for the staining of tubercle bacilli, but the original method as employed by Koch is so satisfactory in its results that it is not advisable to substitute others for it. The above differs from the original Koch-Ehrlich method for the staining of tubercle bacilli in sputum only in the occasional employment of Ziehl's carbolic-fuchsin solution and the method of heating the preparation with the staining fluid upon it.

As Nuttall has pointed out, however, the strong acid decolorizer used in this method can be with advantage replaced by much more dilute solutions, as a certain number of the bacilli are entirely decolorized by the too energetic action of the strong acids. He recommends the following method of decolorization: After staining the slip or section in the usual way, pass it through three alcohols; it is then to be washed out in a solution composed of

> Water . . . . . . 150 c.c.
> Alcohol . . . . . . 50 c.c.
> Concen. sulphuric acid . . . 20 to 30 drops.

From this they are removed to water and carefully rinsed. The remaining steps in the process are the same as those given in the other methods.

GRAM'S METHOD.—Another differential method of staining which is very commonly employed is that known as Gram's method. In this method the objects to be stained are treated with an aniline-water solution of gentian-violet made after the formula of Koch-Ehrlich. After remaining in this for twenty to thirty minutes they are immersed in an iodine solution composed of

> Iodine . . . . 1 gramme.
> Potassium iodide . . . . . 2 grammes.
> Distilled water . . . . . 300 c.c.

In this they remain for about five minutes; they are then transferred to alcohol and thoroughly rinsed. If they are still of a violet color they are again treated with the iodine solution followed by alcohol, and this is continued until no trace of violet color is visible to the naked eye. They may then be examined, or a contrast color of carmine or Bismarck-brown may be given them.

This method is particularly useful in demonstrating the capsule which is seen to surround some bacteria, particularly the diplococcus of pneumonia.

GLACIAL ACETIC ACID METHOD.—Another method which may be employed for demonstrating the presence of the capsule which surrounds certain organisms, is to prepare the cover-slips in the ordinary way, then cover the layer of bacteria upon them with glacial acetic acid, which is instantly poured off (not washed off in water), and the aniline-water gentian-violet solution dropped upon them; this is allowed to remain three or four minutes, is poured off, and again a few drops added, and lastly the slip is washed off in water. A very clear, sharply-cut picture usually follows this method of procedure.

STAINING OF SPORES.—We have learned that one of the points by which spores may be recognized is their refusal to take up staining substances when applied in the ordinary way. They may, however, be stained by special methods; of these the following will prove useful: The cover-slip is to be prepared from the material containing the spores in the ordinary way, dried, and fixed. It is then floated, bacteria down, upon the surface of a watch-crystalful of freshly prepared Koch-Ehrlich solution of fuchsin. This is then held by its edge with the forceps about 2 cm. above a very small flame of a Bunsen burner, care being given that the flame touches only the centre of the bottom of the crystal. After a few seconds the crystal is elevated gradually until it is about 6 to 8 cm. above the flame, then it is slowly moved down to the flame again, and this up-and-down movement is continued until the staining fluid begins to boil. As soon as a few bubbles have been given off it is held aside for a minute or two and the process of heating is repeated. When the boiling begins, again the crystal is held aside for a minute or two. The crystal is heated in this way for about five or six consecutive times. When the fluid has stood for about five minutes after the last boiling, the preparation is transferred, without washing in water, into a second watch-crystal containing the following decolorizing solution:

Absolute alcohol . . . . . . 100 c.c.
Hydrochloric acid . . . . . . 3 c.c.

In this solution it is placed, bacteria up, and the vessel is tilted from side to side for about one minute. It is then removed, washed in water, and stained with the methylene-blue solution. The spores will be stained red and the body of the cells will be blue.

MOELLER'S METHOD FOR STAINING SPORES.—A method that has recently been published by Moeller is designed to favor the penetration of the coloring material through the spore membrane by macerating the spores in a solution of chromic acid before staining them. It is as follows:

The cover-slips are prepared in the usual way, or the fixing may be accomplished with absolute alcohol instead of high temperatures. The preparation is then held for two minutes in chloroform, then washed off in water, then placed for from one-half to two minutes in a 5 per cent. solution of chromic acid; again washed off in water, and now stained in carbolic fuchsin. In the process of staining, the slip is taken by the corner with the forceps and carbolic fuchsin is dropped upon the side containing the spores. It is then held over the flame until it boils, and then held some distance above the flame for one minute. The staining fluid is then poured off and the preparation is completely decolorized in 5 per cent. sulphuric acid, again washed off in water, and finally stained for thirty seconds in the watery methylene-blue solution. The spores will be red, the body of the cells blue.

In this method the object of the preliminary exposure to chloroform is to dissolve away any crystals of lecithin, cholesterin, or fat that may be in the preparation, and which when stained might give rise to confusion.

LÖFFLER'S METHOD FOR STAINING FLAGELLÆ.— For the demonstration of the locomotive apparatus possessed by motile bacteria we are indebted to Löffler. By a special method of staining in which the use of mordants played the essential part, he has shown that these organisms possess very delicate, hair-like appendages, by the lashing movements of which they propel themselves through the fluid in which they are located. The method of Löffler is as follows:

(1) It is essential that the bacteria be evenly and *not too numerously* distributed upon the cover-slip. The slips must therefore be carefully cleansed. (See *Löffler's method* of cleaning cover slips.) Five or six of the carefully cleansed cover-slips are to be placed in a line on the table, and on the centre of each slip a very small drop of tap-water is placed. From the culture to be examined a minute portion is transferred to the first slip and carefully mixed with the drop of water; from this mixture a small portion is transferred to the second, and from the second to the third slip, and so on—in this way insuring a dilution of the number of organisms present in the preparation.

These slips are then dried and fixed in the ordinary way. They are next to be warmed in the following solution:

Tannic acid solution in water (20 acid, 80 water) . . . . 10 c.c.
Cold saturated solution of ferro-sulphate . 5 c.c.
Saturated watery or alcoholic solution of fuchsin . . . . 1 c.c.

This solution represents the mordant. A few drops of it are to be placed upon the film of bacteria on the cover-slip, which is then to be held over the flame until the solution begins to steam. It should not be boiled. After steaming, the mordant is washed off in water and finally in alcohol. The bacteria are to be stained in a saturated aniline-water fuchsin solution.

When treated in this way different bacteria behave differently: the flagellæ of some stain readily in the above solutions; others require the addition of an alkali in varying quantities; while others stain best after the addition of acids. To meet these conditions an exact 1 per cent. solution of caustic soda in water must be prepared, and also a solution of sulphuric acid in water of such strength that one cubic centimentre will be exactly neutralized by one cubic centimetre of the alkaline solution.

For different bacteria which have been studied by this method, the one or the other of these solutions is to be added to the mordant in the following proportions.

Of the acid solution:

For the bacillus of Asiatic cholera . . ½ to 1 drop.
For the spirillum rubrum . . . 9 drops.

Of the alkaline solution:

For the bacillus of typhoid fever . . 1 c.c.
For the bacillus subtilis . . . 28 to 30 drops.
For the bacillus of malignant œdema . 36 to 37 "

For other organisms one must determine whether the results are better after the addition of acid or alkali, and how much of either is required. In general it may be said that bacteria which produce acids in the media in which they are growing require the addition of alkalies to the mordant, while those that produce alkalies require acids to be added. By following Löffler's directions the delicate, hair-like flagellæ on motile organisms may be rendered plainly visible.

STAINING IN GENERAL.

The physics of staining and decolorization is hardly a subject to be discussed in a book of this character, but, as Kühne has pointed out, solutions which favor the production of diffusion currents facilitate intensity of staining and by a similar process increase the energy of decolorizing agents. For example, tissues which are transferred from water into watery solutions of the coloring matters are less intensely stained and more easily decolorized than when transferred from alcohol into watery staining fluids; for the same reason tissues stained in watery solutions of the dyes do not become decolorized so readily when placed in water as when placed in alcohol.

The diffusion of staining solutions into the protoplasm of dried bacteria, as found upon cover-slip preparations, is much greater and more rapid than when the same bacteria are located in the interstices of tissues. These differences are not in the bacteria themselves, but in the obstruction to diffusion offered by the tissues in which they are located.

The result of absence of diffusion may easily be illustrated. Prepare a cover-slip preparation, dry it carefully, fix it, and without allowing water to get upon it from any source, attempt to stain it with a solution of the dyes in *absolute alcohol*. The result is negative. The absolute alcohol does not possess the property of diffusing into the dried tissues, and hence, as has been stated before, alcoholic solutions of the staining dyes should not be employed. The staining dyes should always be watery.[1]

DECOLORIZING SOLUTIONS.—As regards the employment of decolorizing agents, it must always be borne in mind that objects which are easily stained are also easily decolorized, and those that can be caused to take up the staining material only with difficulty are also very difficult to rob of their color. The most common decolorizer in use is probably alcohol—not absolute alcohol, but alcohol containing more or less of water. Water alone has this property, but in a much lower degree than dilute alcohol. On the other hand, a much more energetic decolorization than that possessed by either alone can be obtained by alternate exposures to alcohol and water. More energetic in their decolorizing action than either water or alcohol, are solutions of the acids. They appear, particularly when they are alcoholic solutions, to diffuse rapidly into tissues and bacteria and very quickly extract the staining materials which have been deposited there. For this reason these solutions should be employed with much care.

[1] In the beginning of this chapter it was stated that the saturated alcoholic solutions of the dyes do not serve as stains for bacteria. It must be remembered that this holds only when absolute alcohol and perfectly dry coloring matters have been used. If but a small proportion of water is present, the bacteria may be stained with these solutions.

Very dilute acetic acid robs tissues and bacteria of their staining with remarkable activity; still more energetic are solutions of the mineral acids, and particularly, as has been said, when this action is accompanied by the decolorizing properties of alcohol.

The acid solutions that are commonly employed are:

Acetic acid in 0.1 per cent. to 5 per cent. watery solution.

Nitric acid in 20 per cent. to 30 per cent. watery solution.

Hydrochloric acid in 3 per cent. solution in alcohol.

STAINING OF BACTERIA IN TISSUES.

In staining tissues for the purpose of demonstrating the bacteria which they may contain, a number of points must be borne in mind: the conditions which favor the diffusion of the staining fluids into the bacteria are now not so favorable to a rapid staining as they were when the bacteria alone were present upon cover-slips; the staining of tissues therefore requires a longer exposure to the dyes than with the cover-slips. In tissues, too, there are other substances beside the bacteria which become stained, and these, unless robbed in whole or in part of their color, may so mask the stained bacteria as to render them difficult, if not impossible of detection. Tissues must therefore always be subjected to some degree of decolorization, and this must be practised without depriving the bacteria of their color.

The details of the methods of decolorization will be described in the section on the technique of staining.

Another point to be remembered in staining tissues is that they can never be heated and retain their structure, in the same way that one heats cover-slips. The best results are not obtained in efforts to hasten the staining by subjection to high temperatures, but rather by longer exposures at lower temperatures.

HARDENING THE TISSUES.—The bits of tissue—not greater than 1 cm. cube—are to be placed, as fresh as possible, in absolute alcohol. The bit of tissue should rest upon a pad of cotton or filter-paper in the bottle containing the alcohol, in order that it may be elevated and surrounded by the part of the alcohol which is specifically the lightest, and consequently contains least water. The alcohol abstracts water from the tissue, and, as the dehydration proceeds, the tissue becomes accordingly more and more dense. When of about the consistency of fresh solid rubber, or preferably not quite so dense, it is ready to cut. A small portion of about 0.5 cm. cube should be cemented to a bit of cork with ordinary mucilage, and allowed to remain in the open air for a minute or two for the mucilage to harden. Alcohol should be dropped upon it occasionally, to prevent drying of the tissue. When the mucilage is hard, the cork with the piece of tissue upon it may be left in alcohol over night, and on the following day it may be cut.

SECTION-CUTTING.—This is accomplished by the use of an instrument known as a microtome (Fig. 22). It is an apparatus provided with a clamp for holding the cork upon which the tissue is cemented and also a sliding clamp which carries a knife. The tissue is clamped horizontally, and the knife is caused to slide across its upper surface, also in the horizontal direction. Beneath the clamp for holding the tissue is a milled disc, by means of which a screw is caused to revolve, and in revolving raises or lowers the clamp holding the tissue, so that the tissue may be brought closer to or farther from the plane in which the knife slides. By this arrangement sections of any desired thickness can be cut by turning the milled disc with the one hand and causing the knife to traverse the tissue with the other.

The tissue and the knife-blade should be kept wet with alcohol, so that the sections may float upon the blade of the knife, from which they can be easily removed without tearing, with a curved needle or a camel-hair pencil. As the sections are cut they are placed in a dish containing alcohol.

Fig. 22.

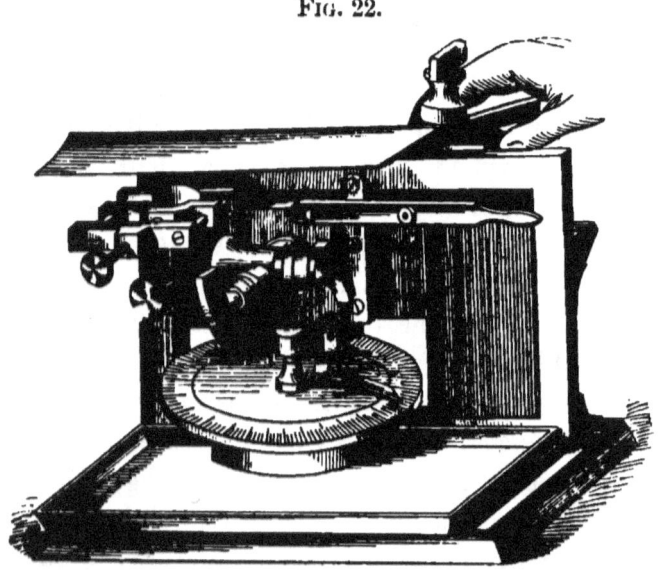

There are some tissues which, by reason of their histological structure, do not become sufficiently dense when exposed to alcohol to permit of their being cut in the above way. It becomes necessary to render them more solid by filling their interstices with some substance that neither interferes with their structure nor prevents their being cut into sections. They must be "imbedded," as this process is called.

Imbedding in celloidin. Most convenient for this purpose is celloidin, a body somewhat similar to collodion, soluble in a mixture of equal parts of alcohol and ether, as well as in absolute alcohol.

Two solutions of celloidin are to be employed, the one a thin solution in a mixture of absolute alcohol and ether, equal parts, the other a thick solution in absolute alcohol. Into the thin solution the tissue is placed from absolute alcohol, and allowed to remain for twenty-four or forty-eight hours. It is then placed in the thick solution for one or two days. From this it may be removed and placed immediately upon a bit of cork. The adherent celloidin will act as a cement, and as it hardens rapidly, the tissue is soon fast to the cork; after remaining in 60 per cent. alcohol for twenty-four hours to complete the solidification of the celloidin, sections may be cut as in the way just described for tissues not so treated.

The paraffin method of imbedding is not to be recommended for bacteriological purposes.

STAINING OF THE SECTIONS.—The sections when cut may be stained in a variety of ways. The ordinary watery solutions of the three common basic aniline dyes —fuchsin, gentian-violet, or methylene-blue—or, what is better, the alkaline methylene-blue solution of Löffler, may be employed for general use.

The acid aniline dyes, as well as some of the vegetable coloring matters, are essentially nuclear stains, and are not applicable to the staining of bacteria.

Into a watch-glass containing either of the staining

solutions mentioned, the sections are to be placed after having been in water for about one minute. They remain in the staining solutions for from five to eight minutes. They are then removed, rinsed in water, and partly decolorized in 0.1 per cent. acetic acid for only a few seconds; again washed out in water, then in absolute alcohol for a few seconds, and from this again into absolute alcohol for the same time, and finally into cedar oil or xylol. Here they remain for from one-half to three-fourths of a minute. They are now to be carefully spread out upon a spatula, which is held in the fluid under them, and without draining off the fluid are transferred to a clean glass slide. This must be done carefully to avoid tearing The easiest way to do this is to hold the spatula on which the section floats in one hand, with its point just touching the surface of the glass slide, and then with a needle pull the section gently off upon the slide. The fluid comes with it, and the floating section may be easily spread out into a flat surface. The excess of fluid is taken up with blotting-paper, after which a drop of xylol-balsam is placed upon the centre of the section, and is then covered with a thin, clean cover-slip. It is now ready for examination.

Each step in the above process has its definite object. The sections are placed in water before staining in order that the diffusion of the staining solution into the tissues may be diminished; otherwise our efforts at rendering the bacteria more conspicuous by decolorizing the tissues in which they are located would rob the bacteria of their color as well.

The acetic acid and also the alcohol are decolorizers, and are directed toward the excess of staining in the tissues. The cedar oil or xylol are bodies which mix on the one hand with alcohol, on the other with balsam.

They are known as "clearing fluids," and fill up the gap that would otherwise be left in the process, for a section cannot be mounted in balsam directly from alcohol; the two bodies do not mix perfectly.

A number of clearing agents are in general use; in fact, almost all the essential oils come under this head. There is one—oil of cloves—which is very commonly used in histological work, but it must not be employed in tissues containing bacteria. It not only extracts too much color from the bacteria, but causes them to fade after the sections have been mounted for a time.

When the section thus stained and mounted is examined microscopically, it may be found that the tissues still possess so much color that the bacteria are not visible, in which case they have not been decolorized sufficiently; or, on the other hand, both bacteria and tissues may have parted with their stains—then decolorization has been carried too far. In either case the fault must be remedied in the manipulation of the next section to be mounted.

In short, the steps in the process of staining sections in general are these:

a. From alcohol into distilled water for one minute.

b. Into the staining fluid for from five to eight minutes.

c. Into water for from three to five minutes.

d. Into 0.1 per cent. acetic acid for about one-half minute.

e. Absolute alcohol for a few seconds.

f. Absolute alcohol for a few seconds.

g. Xylol for about one-half minute.

h. Removal with spatula or section-lifter to slide.

i. Removal of excess of xylol.

j. Mounting in xylol-balsam.

The section must be lifted from one vessel to the other by means of either a curved needle or a glass rod drawn out to a fine end and bent in the form of a curved needle.

By the above process of staining, which can be practised as a general method for most bacteria in tissues, the nuclei of the tissue cells, as well as the bacteria, will be more or less deeply stained.

SPECIAL METHODS OF STAINING BACTERIA IN TISSUES.—For purposes of contrast stains it sometimes becomes necessary to completely, or nearly completely, decolorize the tissues and leave the bacteria unaltered in color. For this purpose special methods depending on the staining peculiarities of the bacteria under consideration have been devised.

Gram's method with tissues. One of the most commonly employed differential stains is that of Gram. In general, it is practised in the way given for its employment on cover-slip preparations with some slight modifications.

In this method the sections are to be placed from water into a solution of aniline-water gentian-violet, as prepared by the Koch-Ehrlich formula, but which has been diluted with about one-third its volume of water. In this the sections remain for about ten minutes, preferably in a warm place, at a temperature of about 40° C. They should never, under any conditions, be boiled.

From this they are washed alternately in the iodine solution and alcohol, occasionally renewing the stained with clean alcohol, until all color has been extracted from them. They are then brought for one minute into a dilute watery solution of eosin or safranin or into picro-carmine; again washed out for a few seconds in alcohol, and finally for one-fourth minute in absolute alcohol.

From this they are transferred to xylol for a half-minute. The remaining steps in the process are the same as those given in the general method. In some cases better results are obtained by reversing the steps in the process and staining the bacteria last, for then the frequent decolorizing action of the alcohol on the bacteria is diminished; thus, place the sections from alcohol into picro-carmine for one-half hour, then wash out in 50 per cent. alcohol, then for from three to five minutes in the dilute aniline-water gentian-violet solution, then into the iodine bath, after three minutes wash out in alcohol, and, finally, for one-fourth minute in absolute alcohol, and then into the xylol, from which they may be mounted. The organisms which may be stained by this method are mic. tetragenus, b. diphtheriæ, b. anthracis, staph. pyogenes aureus, and a few others. It cannot be successfully employed with the bacillus of typhoid fever.

Staining with dahlia and decolorizing with soda solution. Another method that is not very commonly employed, though the results obtained by its use are in many cases very satisfactory, is to stain the tissues in a strong watery solution of dahlia (about one-fourth saturated) for from ten to fifteen minutes; from this they are brought into a two per cent. solution of sodium or potassium carbonate, and from this into alcohol, alternating from the one to the other, until the section is almost colorless. From the alcohol they are rinsed out in water and then brought into a dilute watery solution of either eosin, Bismarck-brown, or safranin for one minute, then washed out in alcohol, finally into absolute alcohol, and then into xylol, from which they may be mounted in the manner given.

Especially brilliant results are obtained when tissues containing anthrax bacilli are stained by this process; the bacilli will be of a deep-blue color, while the surrounding tissues will be of the color used as contrast.

Kühne's carbolic methylene-blue method. Stain the sections in the following solution for from one-half to one hour:

> Methylene-blue, in substance . . 1.5 grammes.
> Absolute alcohol . . . . . 10 c.c.

Rub up thoroughly in a mortar, and when the blue is completely dissolved, add gradually 100 c.c. of a 5 per cent. solution of carbolic acid. (The solution decomposes after a short time; it should be made fresh when needed.) From this the sections are washed out in water, then in 1.5 to 2 per cent. hydrochloric acid in water, from this into a solution of lithium carbonate of the strength of six to eight drops of a concentrated watery solution of the salt to ten drops of water, and from this again thoroughly washed in water; then into absolute alcohol containing enough methylene-blue in substance to give it a tolerably dense color, then for a few minutes into aniline oil to which a little methylene-blue in substance has been added; then completely rinse out in pure aniline oil, from this into thymol or oil of turpentine for two minutes, and then into xylol, from which they are mounted in xylol-balsam. The advantages of this method are that it is generally applicable, and by its use the bacteria are not robbed of their color, whereas the tissues are sufficiently decolorized to render the bacteria visible and admit of the use of contrast stains.

Weigert's modification of Gram's method for sections. Stain the sections in Ehrlich's aniline-water gentian-violet solution for five or six minutes; wash out in water or physiological salt solution (0.6 to 0.7 per cent. solution of sodium chloride in distilled water); transfer them with the section-lifter to the slide; take up the excess of fluid by gently pressing upon the flat section with blotting-paper; treat the section with the iodine solution used by Gram; take up the excess of the solution with blotting-paper; cover the section with aniline oil— this not only differentiates the component parts of the section, but dehydrates as well; wash out the aniline oil with xylol, and mount in the usual way in xylol-balsam. Or, decolorization with iodine may be omitted, and the sections, after staining in the aniline-water gentian-violet for five or six minutes or longer, if necessary, are transferred to the slide without being washed in water or salt solution, or if so only very slightly and rapidly, dried as completely as possible with filter-paper, then are decolorized with a mixture of aniline oil (one part) and xylol (two parts). This is the delicate part of the process and can be watched under the low power of the microscope; when decolorization is sufficient (repeated applications of the aniline oil and xylol mixture are generally necessary), pure xylol replaces the mixture, and the specimen is finally mounted in xylol balsam. Unless all the aniline oil is replaced by the xylol the specimen will not keep well. In this process the aniline oil is really the decolorizer and has the valuable property of absorbing a certain amount of water, so that dehydration with alcohol is avoided. This method, while it stains certain bacteria in tissues very satisfactorily, is nevertheless designed especially for the staining of fibrin. Fibrin and hyaline materal will be stained deep blue, bacteria a dark violet.

150　　　　　　BACTERIOLOGY.

STAINING FOR TUBERCLE BACILLI IN TISSUES.—As for the staining of cover-slips, only those methods most commonly employed will be given.

The method of Ehrlich. Stain the sections in aniline-water fuchsin or gentian-violet for twenty-four hours; decolorize in 20 per cent. nitric acid for a few seconds only, the color need not be entirely extracted; then into 70 per cent. alcohol until no more color can be extracted by the alcohol; stain as contrast color in dilute watery methylene-blue, malachite-green, or Bismarck-brown solution; wash out in 90 per cent. alcohol, then in absolute alcohol for a few seconds; clear up in xylol and mount in xylol-balsam.

Method of Ziehl-Neelsen. Stain the sections in warmed carbol-fuchsin solution for one hour; temperature to be about 45° to 50° C. Decolorize for a few seconds in 5 per cent. sulphuric acid, then in 70 per cent. alcohol, and from this on as by the Ehrlich method.

Dry method. For the tubercle bacilli, as for many other organisms in tissues, the following method may be employed if only the presence of organisms is to be detected and the histological condition of the tissues is a matter of no consequence: Bring the sections from water upon a slide or cover-slip, dry, fix, and stain by the methods for cover-slip preparations.

CHAPTER XIII.

Inoculation of animals—Subcutaneous inoculation, intra-venous injection.

AFTER subjecting an organism to the methods of study that we have just reviewed, it remains that its action upon the lower animals should be tested—*i. e.*, to determine if it possesses the property of producing disease or not, and if so, what are the pathological results of its growth in the tissues of these animals, and in what way must it gain entrance to the tissues in order to produce these results.

This is commonly determined by both subcutaneous and intra-venous inoculation.

SUBCUTANEOUS INOCULATION OF ANIMALS.—The animals usually employed in the laboratory for purposes of inoculation are white mice, gray house-mice, guinea-pigs, rabbits, and pigeons.

For simple subcutaneous inoculation the steps in the process are practically the same in all cases. The hair or feathers are to be carefully removed. If the skin is very dirty it may be scrubbed with soap and water. Disinfection of the skin is impossible, so that it need not be attempted. If the inoculation is to be by means of a hypodermatic syringe, then a fold of the skin may be lifted up and the needle inserted in the way common to this procedure. If a solid culture is to be inoculated, a fold of the skin may be taken up with the forceps and a pocket cut into it with scissors which have previously been sterilized. This pocket must be cut large enough to admit the end of the needle without its touching the sides of the opening as it is inserted. Beneath the skin will be found the superficial and deep connective-tissue fasciæ. These must be taken up with sterilized forceps and with sterilized scissors, and incised in a way corresponding to the skin. The pocket is then to be held open with the forceps and the substance to be inserted is introduced as far back under the skin and fasciæ as possible, care being taken not to touch the edges of the wound if it can be avoided. The wound may be then simply pulled together and allowed to remain. No stitching or efforts at closing it are necessary.

During manipulation the animal must be held quiet. For this purpose special forms of holders have been devised, but if an assistant is to be obtained for the operation, the simple subcutaneous inoculation may be made without the aid of a mechanical holder.

For mice, however, a holder is of much convenience. This piece of apparatus consists of a bit of board of about 7 x 10 cm. and 2 cm. thick, upon which is tacked a hollow, tapering roll of wire gauze, a truncated cone of about 6 cm. long and of about 1.5 cm. in diameter at one end and 2 cm. at its other end.

This is tacked upon the board in such a position that its long axis runs in the long diameter of the board, being equidistant from its two sides. Its small end is placed at the edge of the board. The mouse is taken up by the tail by means of a pair of tongs and allowed to crawl into the smaller end of this wire cone. When so far in that only the root of the tail projects, the animal is then fixed in this position by a clamp and thumb-screw, with which the apparatus (Fig. 23) is provided. The animal usually remains perfectly quiet and may be handled without difficulty.

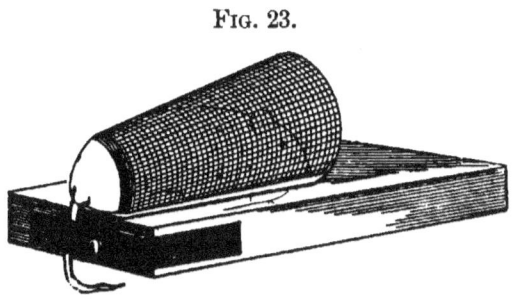

FIG. 23.

The hair from over the root of the tail is to be carefully cut away with the scissors and a pocket cut through the skin at this point. The inoculation is then made into the loose tissues under the skin over this part of the back in the same way that has just been described. It is best always to insert the needle some distance along the spinal column and thus deposit the material as far from the surface-wound as possible.

As the subcutaneous operation is very simple and takes only a few moments, guinea-pigs, rabbits, and pigeons are best held by an assistant. The front legs in the one hand and the hind legs in the other, with the animal stretched upon its back on a table, is the usual position for the operation when practised upon guinea-pigs and rabbits. The point at which the inoculations are commonly made is in the abdominal walls either to the right or left of the median line and about 3 cm. distant. When pigeons are used they are held with the legs, tail, and ends of the wings in the one hand, and the head and anterior portion of the body in the other, leaving the area occupied by the pectoral muscles, over which the inoculation is to be made, free for manipulation. The hair should be closely cut with the scissors in the case of the guinea-pigs and rabbits, and the feathers pulled out in the case of the pigeon.

INJECTION INTO THE CIRCULATION.—It is not infrequently desirable to inject the material under consideration directly into the circulation of an animal. If the rabbit is to be employed for the purpose, the operation is usually done upon one of the veins in the ear.

To those who have had no practice in this procedure it offers a great many difficulties; but if the directions which will be given be strictly observed, the greatest of these obstacles to the successful performance of the operation may be overcome.

When viewing the circulation in the ear of the rabbit by transmitted light, three conspicuous branches of the main vessel (vena auricularis posterior) will be seen. One runs about centrally in the long axis of the ear, one runs along its anterior margin, and one along its posterior margin. The central branch (the ramus anterior of the vena auricularis posterior) is the largest and most conspicuous vessel of the ear, and is, therefore, selected by the inexperienced as the branch into which it would appear easiest to insert a hypodermatic needle. This, however, is fallacious. This vessel lies very loosely imbedded in connective tissue, and in efforts to introduce a needle into it, rolls about to such an extent that only after a great deal of difficulty does the experiment succeed. On the other hand, the posterior branch (ramus lateralis posterior of the vena auricularis posterior) is a very fine, delicate vessel which runs along the posterior margin of the ear, and which is so firmly fixed in the dense tissues which surround it that it is prevented from rolling about under the point of the needle. The further away from the mouth of the vessel—that is, the nearer we approach its capillary extremity—the more favorable become the conditions for the success of the operation.

Select, then, the very delicate vessel lying quite close to the posterior margin of the ear, and make the injection as near to the apex of the ear as possible. The injection is always to be made from the dorsal surface of the ear.

Of no less importance than the selection of the proper vessel, is the shape of the point of the needle employed.

The hypodermatic needles as they come from the makers are not suited at all for this operation because of the way in which their points are ground. If one examines carefully the point of a new hypodermatic needle it will be seen that the long point, instead of presenting a *flat*, slanting surface, when viewed from the side, is more or less of a *curved* surface. Now, in efforts to introduce such a needle into vessel a of very small calibre, it is commonly seen that the extreme point of the needle, instead of remaining in the vessel as it would do were it straight, very commonly projects into the opposite wall, and as the needle is inserted further and further into the tissues, it is usually pushed through the vessels into the loose tissues beyond, and the material to be injected is deposited into these tissues instead of into the circulation. If, on the contrary, the slanting point of the needle is ground down until its surface is perfectly flat, and when viewed from the side no more curvature exists, then when once inserted into a vessel it usually remains there, and there is no tendency to penetrate through the opposite wall. We never use a new hypodermatic needle until its point is carefully ground down to a perfectly flat, slanting surface and no more curvature exists.

These differences may perhaps come out clearer if represented diagrammatically.

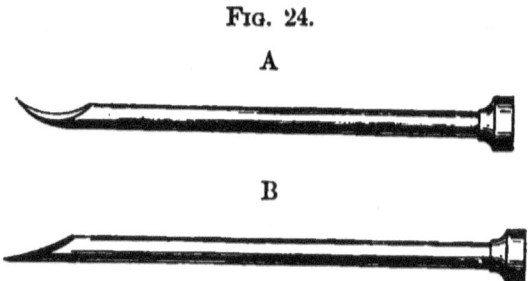

Fig. 24.

In Fig. 24, A, the needle has the point usually seen when new.

In Fig. 24, B, the point has been ground down to the shape best suited for this operation.

The needles need not be returned to the maker. One can grind them to the shape desired in a few minutes upon an oilstone.

The size of the needle is that commonly employed for subcutaneous injections.

When the operation is to be performed, an assistant holds the animal gently but firmly in the crouching position upon a table. If the animal does not remain quiet it is best to wrap it in a towel so that nothing but its head protrudes, though in the most cases we have not found this necessary, and particularly if the animal has not been excited prior to the beginning of the operation.

The animal should be placed so that the ear upon

INJECTION INTO THE CIRCULATION. 157

which the operation is to be performed comes between the operator and the source of light. This renders visible by transmitted light not only the coarser vessels of the ear, but also their finer branches. The point at which the injection is to be made is to be shaved clean of hair, by means of a razor and soap.

The filled hypodermatic syringe is taken in one hand and with the other hand the ear is held firmly. The point of the needle is then inserted through the skin and into the finest part of the ramus posterior, the part nearest the apex of the ear. When the point of the needle is in this vessel it gives to the hand a sensation quite different from that felt when it is in the midst of connective tissue. As soon as one thinks the point of the needle is in the vessel, a drop or two of the fluid may be injected from the syringe, and if his suspicions are correct the circulation in the small ramifications and their anastomoses will quickly alter in appearance. Instead of their containing blood, the colorless fluid which is being injected will now be seen to circulate. This must be carefully observed, for sometimes when the needle-point is not actually in the vessel, but is in the lymph-spaces surrounding it, an appearance somewhat similar is to be seen. It may always be differentiated, however, by continuing the injection, when the circulation of clear fluid through the vessels will not only fail to take the place of the circulating blood but there will at the same time appear a localized swelling under the skin about the point of the needle. The needle must then be withdrawn and inserted into the vessel at a point a little nearer to its proximal end.

Care must be given that no air is injected.

The hypodermatic syringe and needle must, previous

to operation, have been carefully sterilized in the steam sterilizer. The animal must be kept under close observation for about an hour after injection.

The form of syringe best suited for this operation is of the ordinary design, but one that permits of thorough sterilization by steam. It should be made of glass and metal, with asbestos packings. The syringes commonly employed are those shown in Fig. 25—*A*, Koch's; *B*, Strohschein's; *C*, Overlack's.

Fig. 25.

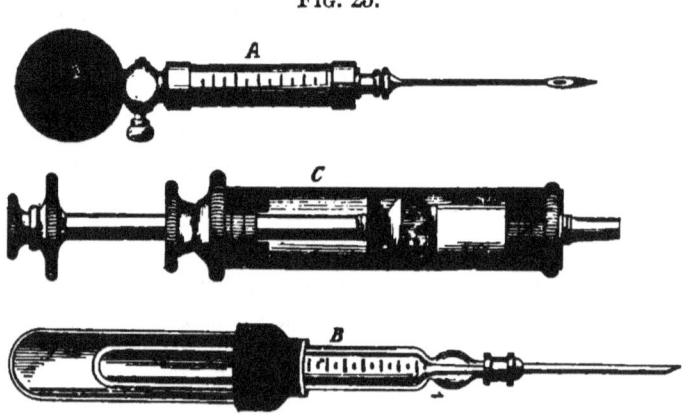

The operation is one that cannot be learned from verbal description. It can only be successfully performed after actual practice.

If the precautions which have been mentioned are observed, but little difficulty in performing the operation will be experienced.

Its convenience and simplicity over other methods for the introduction of substances into the circulation commend it as an operation with which to make oneself familiar. The animals sustain practically no wound, they experience no pain—at least they give no evidence of pain—and no anæsthesia is required.

CHAPTER XIV.

Post-mortem examination of animals—Bacteriological examination of the tissues—Disposal of tissues and disinfection of instruments after the examination.

FOR the purpose of examining bacteriologically the tissues of dead animals, certain rigid precautions must be observed in order to avoid error.

The autopsy should be made as soon as possible after death. If delay cannot be avoided, the animal should be kept on ice until the examination can be made, otherwise decomposition sets in, and the saprophytic bacteria which will now be present may interfere with the accuracy of the results.

When the autopsy is to be made, the animal is first inspected externally, and all visible lesions noted. It is then to be fixed upon its back upon a board with nails or tacks. The four legs and the end of the nose, through which the tacks are driven, are to be moderately extended. The surfaces of the thorax and abdomen are then to be moistened to prevent the fine hairs, dust, etc., from floating about in the air and interfering with the work. An incision is then made through the skin from the chin to the genitalia. This is only a skin incision, and does not reach deeper than the muscles. It is best done by first making a small incision with a scalpel, just large enough to permit of the introduction of one blade of a blunt-pointed scissors. It is then completed with the scissors. The whole of the skin is then carefully dissected away, not only from the abdomen and thorax, but from the axillary, inguinal, and cervical regions, and the fore and hind legs as well. The skin is then pinned back to the board so as to keep it as far from the abdomen and thorax as possible, for it is from the skin that the chances of contamination are greatest.

It now becomes necessary to proceed very carefully. All incisions from this time on are to be made only through surfaces that have been sterilized. This is best accomplished by the use of a broad-bladed common knife which can be heated in the gas-flame. The blade is to be heated quite hot, and is to be held upon the region of the linea alba until the skin at that region begins to burn; it is then held transverse to this line over about the centre of the abdomen, thus making two sterilized tracks through which the abdomen may be opened by a crucial incision. The sterilization thus accomplished is, of course, directed only against organisms that may have fallen upon the surface from without, and it therefore need not extend deep down through the tissues.

In the same way two burned lines may be made from either extremity of the transverse line up to the top of the thorax.

With a hot scissors the central longitudinal incision, extending from the point of the sternum to the genitalia, is to be made without touching the internal viscera. The abdominal wall must therefore be held up during the operation with sterilized forceps or hook.

The cross incision is made in the same way. When this is completed, an incision through the ribs with a pair of heavy scissors, which have been sterilized, is made along the scorched tracks on either side of the thorax.

After this the whole anterior wall of the thorax may

easily be lifted up, and by severing the connections with the diaphragm it may be completely removed.

When this is done and the abdominal flaps laid back, the contents of both cavities are to be inspected and their condition noted without disturbing them.

After this, the first steps to be taken are to prepare plates or Esmarch tubes from the point of inoculation, the blood, liver, spleen, kidneys, and any exudates that may exist.

This is best done as follows:

Heat a scalpel quite hot and apply it to a small surface of the organ from which the cultures are to be made. Hold it upon the organ until the surface directly beneath it is visibly scorched. Then remove it, heat it again and while quite hot insert its point through the capsule of the organ. Into the opening thus made insert a sterilized platinum-wire loop, made of wire a little heavier than that commonly employed. Project this deeply into the tissues of the organ; by twisting it about, enough material from the centre of the organ can be obtained for making plates or Esmarch tubes.

The cultures from the blood are usually made from one of the cavities of the heart, which is always entered through a surface which has been burned in the way given.

In addition to cultures, cover-slips from each organ and from any exudates that may exist, must be made. These, however, are prepared *after* the materials for the cultures have been obtained.

They need not be examined immediately, but may be placed aside, under cover, on bits of paper upon which the name of the organ from which they were prepared is written.

When the autopsy is complete and the gross appearances have been carefully noted, small portions of each organ are to be preserved in 95 per cent. alcohol for subsequent examination. Throughout the entire autopsy it must be borne in mind that all cultures, cover-slips, and tissues must be carefully labelled, not only with the name of the organ from which they originate, but with the date, name of the animal, etc., so that an account of their condition after closer study may be subsequently inserted in the protocol.

The cover-slips are now to be stained, mounted, and examined microscopically, and the results carefully noted in the protocol.

The same may be said for the subsequent study of the cultures and the hardened tissues which are to be stained and subjected to microscopic examination. The results of the microscopic study of the cover-slip preparations and those obtained by cultures should in most cases correspond, though it not rarely occurs that bacteria are present in such small numbers in the tissues that their presence may be overlooked microscopically, and still they may appear in the cultures.

If the autopsy has been performed in the proper way, under the precautions given, and sufficiently soon after death, the results of the bacteriological examination should be either negative or the organisms which appear should be in pure cultures.

This is particularly the case with the cultures made from the internal viscera.

Both the cover-slips and cultures made from the point of inoculation are apt to contain a variety of organisms.

If the organism obtained in pure culture from the internal viscera, or those predominating at the point of inoculation of the animal, have caused its death, then subsequent inoculation of pure cultures of this organism into the tissues of a second animal should produce similar results.

When the autopsy is quite finished, the remainder of the animal should be *burned*, all instruments subjected to either sterilization by steam or boiling for fifteen minutes in 1 to 2 per cent. soda solution, and the board upon which the animal was tacked, as well as the tacks, towels, dishes, and all other implements used at the autopsy, are to be sterilized by steam. All cultures, cover-slips, and indeed, all articles likely to have infectious material upon them, must be thoroughly sterilized as soon as they are of no further service.

CHAPTER XV.

Scheme for the complete study of an organism.

THE following scheme will serve as a guide for the systematic study of an organism :
1. Its form and grouping as seen when discovered.
2. Where discovered.
3. The appearance of its colonies on gelatin plates or Esmarch tubes.
4. The appearance of its colonies on agar-agar plates or Esmarch tubes.
5. The appearance of its growth in stab and slant cultures on gelatin.
6. The appearance of its growth in stab and slant cultures on agar-agar.
7. Its growth on potato.
8. Its growth on blood-serum.
9. Its behavior in bouillon.
10. Its behavior in milk, plain.
11. Its behavior in peptone-rosolic-acid solution.
12. Its behavior in milk containing litmus solution.
13. What is its normal morphology? What morphological changes does it pass through under varying conditions of life?
14. Does it form spores?
15. Is it motile? Are the flagellæ demonstrable by Löffler's method of staining? Is an acid or an alkali to be added to the mordant; if so, the quantity? In

what way are the flagellæ given off from the body of the organism?

16. Does it produce gas-bubbles in ordinary agar-agar or gelatin?

17. Does it produce gas-bubbles in agar-agar or gelatin to which 1 to 2 per cent. grape sugar has been added?

18. Does it produce indol? Is the indol accompanied by a coincident production of nitrites?

19. At what temperature does it grow most luxuriantly?

20. What is the lowest temperature at which it grows?

21. Is it aërobic, anaërobic, or facultative in its relations to oxygen?

22. What are its staining peculiarities?

23. Will it withstand drying?

24. At what temperature is it killed by heat—both by steam and the hot-air method?

25. Is it pathogenic when introduced either subcutaneously or directly into the circulation of animals? If so, for which animals? Do any of the animals used for this work possess natural immunity against infection by this organism?

26. What are the histological appearances seen in the tissues of animals for which this organism is pathogenic?

PRACTICAL APPLICATION OF THE METHODS OF BACTERIOLOGY.

CHAPTER XVI.

To obtain material upon which to begin work.

EXPOSE to the air of an inhabited room a slice of freshly steamed potato or a bit of slightly moistened bread upon a plate for about one hour. Then cover it with an ordinary water-glass and place it in a warm spot (temperature not to exceed that of the human body—37.5° C.), and allow it to remain unmolested. At the end of twenty-four to thirty-six hours there can be seen upon the cut surface of the bread or potato small, round, oval, or irregularly round patches which present various appearances.

These differences in macroscopic appearance consist in some cases in the presence or absence of color; again in a higher or lower degree of moisture; in some instances a patch will be glistening and smooth while its neighbor may be dull and rough or wrinkled. Here will appear an island regularly round in outline and there an area covered by an irregular ragged deposit. All of these gross appearances are of value in aiding us to distinguish between these colonies—for colonies they are—and under the same conditions the organisms composing each of them will always produce growths of exactly the same appearance. It was just such an experiment as this, accidentally performed, that suggested to Koch a means of separating and isolating from mixtures of bacteria the component individuals in pure cultures, and it is upon this observation that the methods of cultivation on solid media are based.

If, without molesting our experiment, we continue the observation from day to day, we may notice changes in the colonies due to the growth and multiplication of the individuals composing them. In some cases the colonies will always retain their sharply cut, round, or oval outline, and will increase but little in size beyond that reached after forty-eight to seventy-two hours, whereas others will spread rapidly, and will very quickly overrun the surface upon which they are growing, and indeed, grow over the smaller, less rapidly developing colonies. In a number of instances, if the observation be continued long enough, many of these rapidly growing colonies will, after a time, lose their lustrous and smooth or regular surface and will show, at first here and there, elevations which will continue to appear until the whole surface takes on a wrinkled appearance. Again bubbles may be seen here and there through the colonies. These are due to the escape of gas resulting from fermentation which the organisms bring about in the medium upon which they are growing. Sometimes peculiar odors resulting from the same cause will be noticed.

Note carefully all these changes and appearances, as they must be employed subsequently in identifying the individual organisms from which each colony on the medium is growing.

If now we examine these points upon our bread or potato with a hand-lens of low magnifying power we will be enabled to detect differences not noticeable to the naked eye. In some cases we shall still see nothing more than a smooth non-characteristic surface; while in others, minute, sometimes regularly arranged corrugations may be observed. In one colony they may appear as tolerably regular radii, radiating from a central spot; and again they may appear as concentric rings; and if by the methods which have been described we obtain from these colonies their individual components in pure culture, we shall see that this characteristic arrangement in folds, radii, or concentric rings, or the production of color, is under normal conditions constant.

So much for the simplest naked-eye experiment that can be made in bacteriology and which serves to furnish the beginner with material upon which to begin his studies. It is not necessary at this time for him to burden his mind with names for these organisms; it is sufficient for him to recognize that they are mostly of different species and that they possess characteristics which will enable him to differentiate the one from the other.

In order now for him to proceed it is necessary that he should have familiarized himself with the methods by which his media are prepared and the means employed in sterilizing them and retaining them sterile—*i. e.*, of preventing the access of foreign germs from without—otherwise his efforts to obtain and retain his organisms as pure cultures will be in vain.

EXPOSURE AND CONTACT.—Make a number of plates from bits of silk used for sutures, after treating them as follows:

Place some of these pieces (about 5 centimetres long) into a sterilized test-tube, and sterilize them by steam for one hour. At the end of the sterilization remove one piece with sterilized forceps and allow it to brush against your clothing, then make a plate from it; another piece draw across the table and then plate it. Suspend upon a sterilized wire hook three or four pieces and let them hang for thirty mintues free in the air, being sure that they touch nothing but the hook; then plate them separately.

Note the results.

In what way do these experiments differ and how can the differences be explained?

Expose to the air six Petri dishes into which either sterilized gelatin or agar-agar has been poured and allowed to solidify; allow them to remain exposed for five, ten, fifteen, twenty, twenty-five, and thirty minutes, in a room where no one is at work. Treat a second set in the same way in a room where several persons are moving about. Be careful that nothing touches them, and that they are exposed only to the air. Each dish must be carefully labled with the time of its exposure.

Do they present different results? What is the reason for this difference?

Which predominate, colonies resulting from the growth of bacteria, or those from common moulds?

How do you account for this condition?

CHAPTER XVII.

Various experiments in sterilization—Steam and hot-air methods of sterilizing.

PLACE in one of the openings in the cover of the steam sterilizer an accurate thermometer; when the steam has been streaming for a minute or two the thermometer will register 100° C.; wrap in a bundle of towels or rags or pack tightly in cotton a maximum thermometer; let this thermometer be in the centre of a bundle large enough to quite fill the chamber of the sterilizer. At the end of a few minutes exposure to the streaming steam remove it; it will be found to indicate a temperature of 100° C.

Closer study of the penetration of steam has taught us, however, that the temperature which is found at the centre of such a mass may sometimes be that of the air in the meshes of the material, and not that of steam, and for this reason the sterilization at that point may not be complete, because hot air at 100° C. has not the destructive properties that steam at the same temperature possesses. It is necessary, therefore, that this air should be expelled from the meshes of the material and its place taken by the steam before sterilization is complete. This is insured by allowing the steam to stream through the substances a few minutes before beginning to calculate the time of exposure. There is as yet no absolutely sure means of saying that the temperature at the centre of the mass is that of hot air or of steam, so that the exact length of time that is required for the expulsion of the air from the meshes of the material cannot be given.

Determine if the maximum thermometer indicates a temperature of 100° C. at the centre of a moist bundle in the same way as when a dry bundle was employed.

To about 50 c.c. of bouillon add about one gramme of chopped hay, and allow it to stand in a warm place for twenty-four hours. At the end of this time it will be found to contain a great variety of organisms. Continue the observation, and a pellicle will be seen to form on the surface of the fluid. This pellicle will be made up of rods which grow as long threads in parallel strands. In many of these rods glistening spores will be seen. After thoroughly shaking, filter the mass through a fine cloth to remove coarser particles.

Pour into each of several test-tubes about 10 c.c. of the filtrate. Allow one tube to remain unmolested in a warm place. Place another in the steam sterilizer for five minutes. A third should remain for ten minutes. A fourth for one-half hour. A fifth for one hour.

At the end of each of these exposures inoculate a tube of sterilized bouillon from each tube. Likewise make a set of plates or Esmarch tubes upon both gelatin and agar-agar from each tube, and note the results. At the same time prepare a set of plates or Esmarch tubes on agar-agar and on gelatin from the tube which has not been exposed to the action of the steam.

The plates or tubes from the unmolested tube will present colonies of a variety of organisms; separate and study these.

Those from the tube which has been sterilized for five minutes will present colonies in moderate numbers, but, as a rule, they will represent but a single organism. Study this organism in pure cultures.

The same may be predicted for the tube which has been heated for ten minutes, though the colonies will be fewer in number.

The thirty-minute tube may or may not give one or two colonies of the same organism.

The tube which has been heated for one hour is usually sterile.

The bouillon tubes from the first and second tubes which were heated will usually show the presence of only one organism—the bacillus which gave rise to the pellicle-formation in our original mixture. This organism is the bacillus subtilis, and will serve to illustrate the difference in resistance toward steam between the vegetative and spore stages of the same organism.

Inoculate about 100 c.c. of sterilized bouillon with a very small quantity of a pure culture of this organism, and allow it to stand in a warm place for about six hours. Now subject this culture to the action of steam for five minutes; it will be seen that sterilization, as a rule, is complete.

Treat in the same way a second flask of bouillon, inoculated in the same way with the same organism, but after having stood in a warm place for from forty-eight to seventy-two hours, that is, until the spores have formed, and it will be found that sterilization is not complete—the spores of this organism have resisted the action of steam for five minutes.

To determine if sterilization is complete always resort to the culture methods, as the macroscopic and microscopic methods are deceptive. Cloudiness of the media or the presence of organisms microscopically does not always signify that the organisms possess the property of life.

Inoculate in the same way a third flask of bouillon with a *very small* drop from one of the old cultures upon which the pellicle has formed; mix it well and subject it to the action of steam for two minutes; then place it to one side for from twenty to twenty-four hours, and again heat for two minutes; allow it to stand for another twenty-four hours, and repeat the process on the third day. No pellicle will be formed, and yet spores were present in the original mixture, and, as we have seen, the spores of this organism are not killed by an exposure of five minutes to the steam. How can this result be accounted for?

Saturate several pieces of cotton thread, each about 2 cm. long, in the original decomposed bouillon, and dry them carefully at the ordinary temperature of the room, then at a little higher temperature—about 40° C.—to complete the process. Regulate the temperature of the hot-air sterilizer for about 100° C., and subject several pieces of this infected and dried thread to this temperature for the same lengths of time that we exposed the same organisms in bouillon to the steam, viz.: five, ten, thirty, and sixty minutes. At the end of each of these periods remove a bit of thread, and prepare a set of plates or Esmarch tubes from it. Are the results analogous to those obtained when steam was employed?

Increase the temperature of the dry sterilizer and repeat the process. Determine the temperature and time necessary for the destruction of these organisms by the dry heat. These threads should not be simply laid upon the bottom of the sterilizer, but should be suspended from a glass rod, which may be placed inside the oven, extending across its top from one side to the other.

Place several of the infected threads in the centre of a bundle of rags. Subject this to a temperature necessary to sterilize the threads by the dry method. Treat another similar bundle to sterilization by steam. In what way do the two processes differ?

CHAPTER XVIII.

Bacteriological study of water, air, and soil—Methods of counting the colonies on the plates—Wolffhügel's counting apparatus—Sedgwick's method.

THE possible spread of infectious diseases by means of water-supplies has formed a topic of discussion by sanitarians for a long time.

The school of Von Pettenkofer has always taken the ground that the appearance and spread of epidemic diseases, of which typhoid fever and Asiatic cholera are types, is due more to alterations in the soil, resulting from fluctuations in the level of the soil-water, than to any part that the drinking-water may play; in opposition to this Koch and his pupils hold that these epidemics can, in most instances, be traced directly to the influence of the water-supply.

The weight of evidence as it now stands favors the opinion that these diseases are frequently the result of imperfections in the supply of water intended for domestic purposes, and there exists sufficient proof of this to necessitate our controlling all such supplies by careful quantitative and qualitative bacteriological analyses.

THE QUALITATIVE BACTERIOLOGICAL ANALYSIS OF WATER.—The qualitative bacteriological analysis of water entails much labor, as it requires that not only all the different species of organism found in the water should be isolated, but that each representative should be subjected to systematic study, and its pathogenic or non-pathogenic properties determined.

ANALYSIS OF WATER. 177

For this purpose the methods for the isolation of individual species, which have already been described, and the means of studying these species when isolated, are indispensable.

For this analysis certain precautions essential to accuracy are always to be observed.

The sample is to be collected under the most rigid precautions that will exclude organisms from sources other than that under consideration. If drawn from a spigot, it should never be collected until the water has been flowing for 15 to 20 minutes in a full stream. If obtained from a stream or a spring, it should be collected, not from the surface, but rather from about one foot beneath the surface.

It should always be collected in vessels which have previously been thoroughly freed from all dirt and organic particles, and then sterilized. And the plates should be made as quickly after collecting the sample as is possible.

Where circumstances permit, all water analyses should be made on the spot at which the sample is taken, as it is known that during transportation, unless the samples are kept packed in ice, a multiplication of the organisms contained in it always occurs.

It is therefore advisable that where this work is to be done, the Esmarch tubes or Petri plates should be prepared on the spot.

For the purpose of qualitative analysis it is necessary that a small portion of the water—one, two, three, five drops—should first be employed as the amounts from which plates are to be made. In this way one forms some idea as to the approximate number of organisms in the water, and can in consequence determine the amount of water necessary to use for each set of plates.

Duplicate plates are always to be made—one set upon agar-agar, which are to be kept at the body-temperature, and one set upon gelatin, which are to be kept at a temperature of 18° to 20° C.

As soon as the colonies have developed, the plates are to be carefully compared and studied. It is to be noted if any difference in the appearance and number of organisms on corresponding plates exist, and if so on which plates the larger number of colonies have developed. In this way the temperature most favorable for the growth of most of these organisms may be determined. The opinion has been advanced that many of the organisms constantly present in water, which make up its normal flora, develop better at a lower than at a higher temperature. This will not be the case, however, if pathogenic forms are present, because they, as a rule, require the body-temperature for their most favorable development, though some of them do grow very well at a lower temperature.

The isolation of the different species and their systematic study is to be conducted in the way given for all bacteria.

THE QUANTITATIVE ESTIMATION OF BACTERIA IN WATER.—The quantitative analysis requires more care in the measurement of the exact volume of water employed, for the results are to be expressed in terms of the number of individual organisms to a definite volume. The necessity for making the plates at the place at which the sample is collected is to be particularly accentuated in this analysis, for the multiplication of the organisms during transit is so great that the results of analyses made after the water has been in a vessel for a day or two are often very different from those which would have been obtained on the spot.

Where it is not possible, however, to make the analysis on the spot, the sample of water should be collected and packed in ice and kept on ice until ready for use, which should in all cases be as soon after its collection as possible.

For the collection of water for this purpose, the best vessel to be employed is a glass bulb (Fig. 26) or balloon, which one soon learns to make for himself from glass tubing.

It consists simply of a round glass sphere blown on the end of a glass tube, which latter is subsequently

Fig. 26.

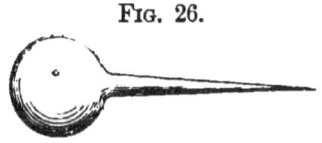

drawn out into a fine capillary stem and sealed while hot. As it cools, the contraction of the air within the bulb results in the production of a negative pressure. If the point of the stem be broken off under water, the bulb is quickly filled because of the existence of the negative pressure within it.

A number of them may be blown, sealed, and kept on hand. They are sterile so long as they are sealed, because of the heat that is employed in their manufacture.

When a sample of water is to be taken, the point of a bulb is simply broken off with sterilized forceps under water at the place from which the sample is to be taken. It rapidly fills with water. This may serve as a sample.

from which to prepare plates or Esmarch tubes on the spot, or the tip of the stem may be re-sealed in the flame of an alcohol lamp, the bulb packed in ice, and transported in this condition to the laboratory.

In beginning the quantitative analysis of water with which one is not acquainted, there are certain preliminary steps that are essential.

It is necessary to know approximately the number of organisms contained in any fixed volume, so as to determine the quantity of water to be employed for the plates or tubes. This is done usually by making preliminary plates from one drop, two drops, 0.25 c.c., 0.5 c.c., and 1 c.c. of the water. After each plate has been labelled with the amount of water used in making it, it is placed aside for development. When this has occurred, one selects the plate upon which the colonies are only moderate in number—about 200 to 300 colonies presenting—and employs in the subsequent analysis the same amount of water that was used in making this plate.

If the original water contained so many organisms that there developed on a plate or tube made with one drop too many colonies to be easily counted, then the sample must be diluted with one, two, or three volumes, as the case may be, of sterilized distilled water. This dilution must be *accurate*, and its exact extent noted, so that subsequently the number of organisms per volume in the original water may be calculated.

The use of a drop is not sufficiently accurate. The dilution should therefore always be to a degree that will admit of the employment of a volume of water that may be exactly measured, 0.25, 0.5 c.c. being the amounts most convenient for use.

COUNTING COLONIES ON PLATES. 181

Duplicate plates should always be made and the mean of the number of colonies that develop upon them taken as the basis from which to calculate the number of organisms per volume in the original water.

For example: From a sample of water, 0.25 c.c. is added to a tube of liquefied gelatin, carefully mixed and poured out as a plate. When development occurs, the number of colonies are too numerous to be accurately counted.

One cubic centimetre of the original water is then to have added to it, under precautions that prevent contamination from without, 99 c.c. of sterilized distilled water—that is, we have now a dilution of 1 : 100. Again, 0.25 c.c. of this dilution is plated and we find 180 colonies on the plate. Assuming that each colony develops from an individual bacterium, though this is perhaps not strictly true, we had 180 organisms in 0.25 c.c. of our 1 : 100 dilution, therefore in 0.25 c.c. of the original water we had $180 \times 100 = 18,000$ bacteria, which will be 72,000 bacteria per cubic centimetre (0.25 = 18,000, 1 c.c. = $18,000 \times 4 = 72,000$). The results are always to be expressed in terms of the number of bacteria per cubic centimetre of the original water.

Throughout this part of the work it is to be borne in mind that when one refers to plates it is not to a set, as in the isolation experiments, but to a single plate.

METHOD OF COUNTING THE COLONIES ON THE PLATES. — For convenience in counting colonies on plates or in tubes, it is of advantage to divide the whole area of the gelatin occupied by colonies into smaller areas of exact size. For this purpose several very convenient devices exist.

182   BACTERIOLOGY.

WOLFFHÜGEL'S COUNTING APPARATUS.—This apparatus (Fig. 27) consists of a flat wooden stand, the

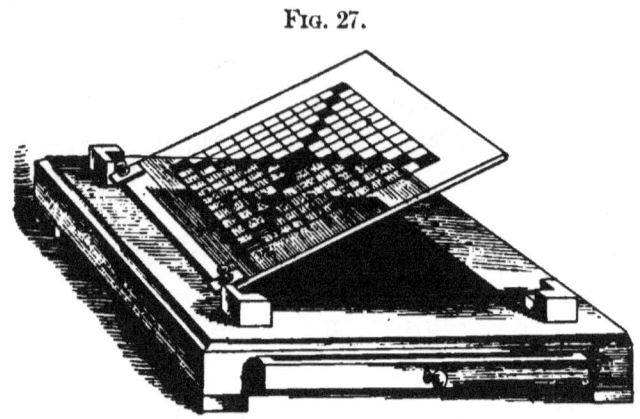

FIG. 27.

centre of which is cut out in such a way that either a black or white glass plate may be placed in it. These form a background upon which the colonies may more easily be seen when the plate to be counted is placed upon it. When the gelatin plate containing the colonies has been placed upon this background of glass, it is then covered by a transparent glass plate which swings on a hinge. When this plate is in position, it is just above the colonies without touching them. This plate is ruled in square centimetres and subdivisions.

The gelatin plate is moved about until it rests under the centre of the area occupied by the ruled lines.

The number of colonies in each square centimetre is then counted, and the sum-total of the colonies in all these areas gives the number of colonies on the plate.

Where the colonies are quite small, as is frequently the case, the counting may be facilitated by the use of a small hand-lens.

In Fig. 28 is seen the form of hand-lens commonly employed.

A plan that is frequently given for the counting of colonies by the use of these devices is to count the number of colonies in each of a number (eight or ten) of the squares, and take the average of these counts as the

FIG. 28.

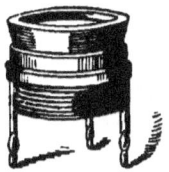

average for each square on the whole surface of the gelatin. The result is then obtained by multiplying this average by the number of squares taken up by the whole surface of the gelatin.

The results vary so much in different counts of the same plate, when made in this way, that they can hardly be considered approximate.

Prepare a plate, calculate the number of colonies upon it by this latter method. Now repeat the calculation making the average from another set of squares. Now actually count the entire number of colonies on the plate. Compare the results.

ESMARCH'S COUNTER.—Esmarch has devised a counter (Fig. 29) for estimating the number of colonies present when they are upon a cylindrical surface, as when in rolled tubes. The principles and methods of estimation are practically the same as those given for Wolffhügel's apparatus. If the number of colonies in an Esmarch tube is to be determined, a simpler method to the use of his apparatus may be employed. It consists in dividing the tube by lines into four or six longitudinal areas which are subdivided by transverse lines drawn about 1 or 2 cm. apart. The lines may be drawn with pen and ink. They need not be exactly the same distance apart,

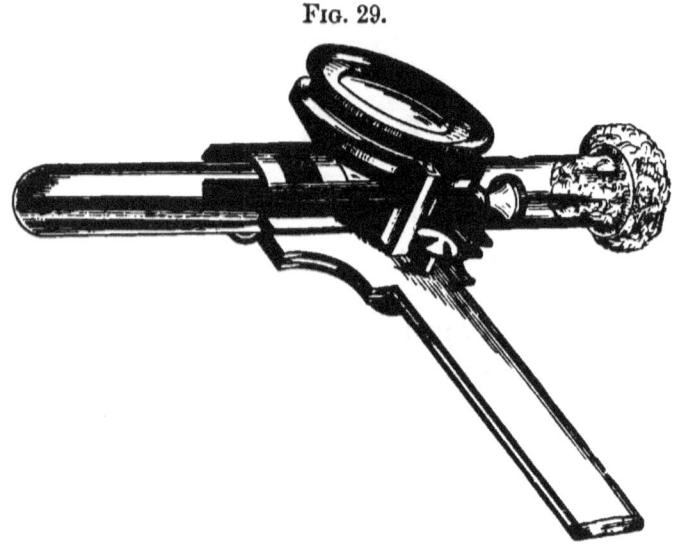

Fig. 29.

or exactly straight. Beginning at one of these squares at one end of the tube, which may be marked with a cross, the tube is twisted with the fingers, always in one direction, and the exact number of colonies in each square as it appears in rotation is counted, care being taken not to count a square more than once; they are then added together, and the result gives the number of colonies in the tube. This method may be facilitated by the use of a hand-lens.

In all these methods there is one error that is difficult to eliminate; it is assumed that each colony represents the outgrowth from a single organism. This is probably not always the case, as there may exist clumps of bacteria which represent hundreds or even thousands of individuals, but which still give rise to but a single colony—this is usually estimated as a single organism in the water under analysis.

Where grounds exist for suspecting the presence of these clumps, they may in part be broken up by shaking the original water with sterilized sand.

What has been said for the bacteriological examination of water, holds good for all fluids which are to be subjected to this form of analysis.

In considering water from a bacteriological standpoint, it must always be borne in mind that comparisons of the water with any general fixed standard are not of much value, for just as normal waters from different sources are seen to present differences in their chemical composition without being unfit for use, so may the number of bacteria per volume in water from one source always be greater or smaller than that from another locality, and yet no differences can be seen to result from their employment. For this reason the proper study of any water, from this point of view, means the establishment of what may be termed its normal proportion of bacteria, as well as a study of the organisms most commonly present. For this purpose experiments covering a long period of time, made at short intervals, must be conducted, and from these observations the means for that water at the different seasons of the year calculated. Marked deviations from these means, either in quantity or quality of the bacteria present, are the only comparisons that are of any value.

A sudden variation from the normal mean in the number of bacteria in any water calls at once for a quantitative chemical analysis as well as a thorough inspection of the supply; at the same time the character of the organisms should be subjected to most careful study.

BACTERIOLOGICAL AIR ANALYSIS.—Quite a number of methods for the bacteriological study of the air exist.

In the main they consist either of allowing air to pass over solid nutrient media (Koch, Hesse) and observing the colonies which develop upon the media, or of filtering the bacteria from the air by means of porous and liquid substances, and studying the organisms thus obtained. (Miguel, Petri, Strauss, Würz, Sedgwick.)

The former methods have given place almost entirely to the latter for reasons of greater exactness possessed by the latter.

In some of the methods which provide for the filtration of bacteria from the air by means of liquid substances, a measured volume of air is aspirated through liquefied gelatin; this is then rolled into an Esmarch tube, and the number of colonies counted, just as was done in the water analysis. This is the simplest procedure. An objection raised against it is that organisms may be lost, and not come into the calculation, by passing through the medium in the centre of an air-bubble without being arrested by the fluid, an objection that appears more of speculative than of real value.

The methods of filtration through porous substances appear, on the whole, to give the best results. Petri recommends the aspiration of a measured volume of air through glass tubes into which sterilized sand is packed. (Fig. 30.) When the aspiration is finished the sand is mixed with liquefied gelatin, plates are made, and the number of developing colonies counted, the results giving the number of organisms contained in the volume of air aspirated through the sand.

FIG. 30.

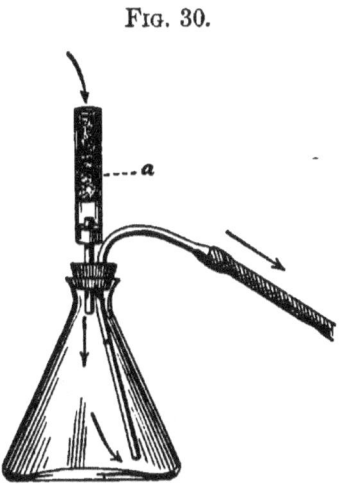

The tube packed with sand is seen at the point *a*.

The main objection to this method is the possibility of mistaking a sand granule for a colony. This objection has been overcome by Sedgwick, who employs granulated sugar instead of the sand; this when brought into the liquefied gelatin dissolves, and no such error as that possible in the Petri method can be made.

SEDGWICK'S METHOD.—On the whole, the method proposed by Sedgwick gives such uniform results that it is to be recommended above the others. It is as follows:

The apparatus employed consists essentially of three parts:

(1) A glass tube of a special form to which the name *aërobioscope* has been given.

(2) A stout copper cylinder of about sixteen litres capacity, provided with a vacuum-gauge.

(3) An air-pump.

The aërobioscope (Fig. 31) is about 35 cm. in its entire length; it is 15 cm. long and 4.5 cm. in diameter at its expanded part; one end of the expanded part is narrowed down to a neck 2.5 cm. in diameter and 2.5 cm. long. To the other end is fused a glass tube 15 cm. long and 0.5 cm. inside diameter, in which is to be placed the filtering material.

FIG. 31.

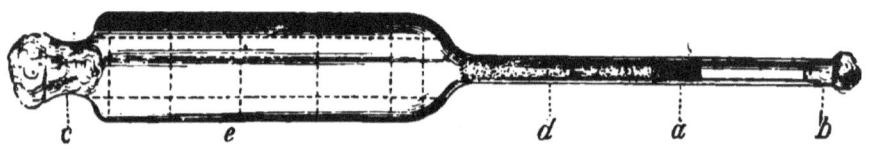

Upon this narrow tube, 5 cm. from the lower end, a mark is made with a file, and up to this mark a small roll of brass-wire gauze (a) is inserted; this serves as a stop for the filtering material which is to be placed over it. Beneath the gauze at (b), and also at the large end (c), the apparatus is plugged with cotton. When thoroughly cleaned, dried, and plugged, the apparatus is to be sterilized in the hot-air sterilizer. When cool, the cotton plug is removed from the large end (c), and sterilized No. 50 granulated sugar is poured in until it just fills the 10 cm. (d) of the narrow tube above the wire gauze. This column of sugar is the filtering material employed to engage and retain the microörganisms. After pouring in the sugar, the cotton-wool plug is replaced, and the tube is again sterilized at 120° C. for several hours.

Taking the air sample. In order to measure the amount of air used, the value of each degree on the vacuum-gauge is determined in terms of air by means of an air-meter, or by calculation from the known capacity of the cylinder. This fact ascertained, the negative pressure indicated by the needle on exhausting the cylinder shows the volume of air which must pass into it in order to fill the vacuum. By means of the air-pump one exhausts the cylinder until the needle reaches the mark corresponding to the amount of air required.

A sterilized aërobioscope is now to be fixed in the upright position and its small end connected by a rubber tube with a stop-cock on the cylinder. The cotton plug is then removed from the upper end of the aërobioscope, and the desired amount of air is aspirated through the sugar. The organisms will be held back by the sugar. During manipulation the cotton plug is to be protected from contamination with germs from without.

When the required amount of air has been aspirated through the sugar the cotton plug is replaced, and by gently tapping the aërobioscope while held in an almost horizontal position, the sugar, and with it the bacteria, are brought into the large part (*e*) of the apparatus. When all the sugar is thus shaken down into this part of the apparatus, about 20 c.c. of liquefied sterilized gelatin is poured in through the opening at the end c, the sugar dissolves, and the whole is then rolled on ice, just as is done in the preparation of an ordinary Esmarch tube.

The gelatin is most easily poured into the aërobioscope by the use of a small, sterilized cylindrical funnel (Fig.

190   BACTERIOLOGY.

32), the stem of which is bent to an angle of about 110° with the long axis of the body.

The larger part of the aërobioscope is divided into squares to facilitate the counting of the colonies. By the employment of this apparatus one can make these analyses at any place, and can, without fear of contamination, carry the tubes to the laboratory, where the cultivation part of the work may be done.

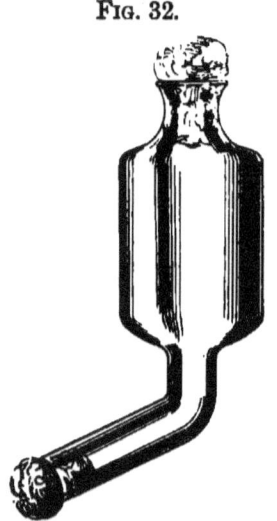

Fig. 32.

Aside from this advantage, the use of a vacuum-cylinder permits a known volume of air to be aspirated with great ease, and its rate of flow through the filter regulated to a nicety.

The filter being soluble, only the insoluble bacteria are left imbedded in the gelatin.

For general use this method is to be preferred to the others that have been mentioned.

BACTERIOLOGICAL STUDY OF THE SOIL.—Bacteriological study of the soil may be made by either breaking up small particles of earth in liquefied media and making plates directly from this, or by what is perhaps a better method, as it gets rid of insoluble particles which may give rise to errors : breaking up the soil for investigation in sterilized water and then making plates from the water.

It must be borne in mind that many of the ground organisms belong to the anaërobic group, so that in these studies this point should be remembered and the methods for the cultivation of these organisms practised in connection with the ordinary methods.

CHAPTER XIX.

Inoculation experiments with sputum—Sputum septicæmia—Septicæmia resulting from the presence of the micrococcus tetragenus in the tissues—Tuberculosis.

OBTAIN from a tuberculous patient a sample of fresh sputum—that of the morning is preferable. Spread it out in a thin layer upon a black glass plate and select one of the small, white, cheesy masses or dense mucous clumps that will be seen scattered through the sputum. With a pointed forceps smear it carefully upon two or three thin cover-slips, dry and fix them in the way given for ordinary cover-slip preparations. Stain one in the ordinary way with Löffler's alkaline methylene-blue solution, the other by the Gram method, the third after the method given for tubercle bacilli in fluids or sputum.

In that stained by Löffler's method—slip No. 1—will be seen a great variety of organisms—round cells, ovals, short and long rods, perhaps spiral forms. But not infrequently will be seen diplococci, having more or less of a lancet shape; they will be joined together by their broad ends, the points of the lancet being away from the point of juncture of the two cells. There may also be seen masses of cocci which are conspicuous for their arrangement into groups of fours, the adjacent surfaces being somewhat flattened. They are not sarcinæ, as one can see by the absence of the division in the third direction—they divide only in two directions.

INOCULATION WITH SPUTUM. 193

In the slip stained by the Gram method the same groups of the cocci which grow as threes and fours will be seen, but our lancet-shaped diplococci will now present an altered appearance—there can now be detected a capsule surrounding them. This capsule is very delicate in structure, and though a frequent accompaniment is not constant. It can sometimes be demonstrated by the ordinary methods of staining, though the method of Gram is most satisfactory.

In the third slip, which has been stained by the method given for tubercle bacilli in sputum, if decolorization has been properly conducted and no contrast stain has been employed, the field will be colorless or of only a very pale rose color. None of the numerous organisms seen in the first slip can now be detected, but instead there will be seen scattered through the field very delicate stained rods, which present, in most instances, a conspicuous beaded arrangement of their protoplasm—that is, the staining is not homogeneous, but at tolerably regular intervals along each rod there is seen alternating intervals of light and color. These rods may be found singly, in groups of twos or threes, or sometimes in clumps consisting of large numbers. When in twos or threes it is not uncommon to find them describing an X or a V in their mode of arrangement, or again they will be seen lying parallel the one to the other.

If contrast stains are used, these rods will be detected and recognized by their retaining the original color with which they have been stained, whereas all other bacteria in the preparation, as well as the tissue-cells which are in the sputum, will take up the contrast color.

These delicate beaded rods are the tubercle bacilli.

The lancet-shaped diplococci with the capsule are the diplococci of sputum septicæmia.

The cocci grouped in fours are the micrococcus tetragenus.

INOCULATION EXPERIMENT.—Inoculate into the subcutaneous tissues of a guinea-pig one of the small white caseous masses similar to that which has been examined microscopically. If death ensues it will be the result of one of the three following forms of infection :

a. Septicæmia[1] resulting from the introduction into the tissues of an organism frequently present in the sputum. It exists under the various names: micrococcus of sputum septicæmia; diplococcus pneumoniæ; pneumococcus of Fränkel; diplococcus lanceolatus—lancet-formed diplococcus; meningococcus; streptococcus lanceolatus Pasteuri.

b. A form of septicæmia resulting from the invasion of the tissues by an organism frequently seen in the sputum of tuberculous subjects. It is characterized by its tendency to divide into fours. It is the micrococcus tetragenus.

c. General or local tuberculosis.

a. SPUTUM SEPTICÆMIA.

If at the end of twenty-four to thirty-six hours the animal is found dead, we may safely suspect that the result was produced by the introduction into the tissues of the organism of sputum septicæmia above mentioned, which is not uncommonly found in the mouth of healthy individuals as well as in other conditions.

[1] Septicæmia is that form of infection in which the blood is the chief field of activity of the organisms.

Inspection reveals nothing abnormal at the seat of inoculation, except when death is postponed for a longer time, when some œdema may be present. At autopsy the most conspicuous naked-eye change will be enlargement of the spleen. Frequently there is a limited fibrinous exudation over portions of the peritoneum.

Except in the exudations, the organisms are found only in the lumen of the bloodvessels, where they are usually present in enormous numbers.

In the blood they are always free and are not found in the body of leucocytes.

In stained preparations from the blood and exudates a capsule is not unfrequently seen surrounding the organisms. This, however, is not constant.

If a drop of blood from this animal be introduced into the tissues of a second animal (mouse, rabbit, or guinea-pig), identically the same conditions will be reproduced.

If the organism be isolated from the blood of the animal in pure culture, and a portion of this culture be introduced into the tissues of a susceptible animal, again we shall see the same pathological picture.

It must be remembered, however, that this organism when cultivated for a time on artificial media rapidly loses its virulent properties. If, therefore, failure to reproduce the disease after inoculation from old cultures should occur, it is, in all probability, due to a disappearance of virulence from the organism.

This organism was discovered by Sternberg in 1880. It was subsequently described by A. Fränkel as the etiological factor in the production of acute fibrinous pneumonia.

It is not uncommonly present in the saliva of healthy

individuals, having been found by Sternberg in the oral cavity of about 20 per cent. of healthy persons examined by him. It is constantly to be detected in the rusty sputum of patients suffering from acute fibrinous pneumonia. Its presence has been detected in the middle ear, in the pericardial sac, in the pleura, in the serous cavities of the brain, and indeed it may probably penetrate from its primary seat in the mouth to almost any of the more distant organs.

The organism is commonly found as a diplococcus, though here and there short chains of four to six individuals joined together may be detected. The morphology of the individual cells is more or less oval, or more strictly speaking, lancet-shaped, for at one end there is commonly a pointed appearance. When joined in pairs the junction is always between the broad ends of the ovals, *never* between the pointed extremities.

In preparations directly from the sputum or from the blood of animals, a delicate capsule may frequently be seen surrounding them. This occurs only in preparations directly from the body and is not seen in preparations from cultures.

This organism grows under artificial conditions very slowly, and frequently not at all.

When successfully grown upon the different media it presents somewhat the following appearance:

On gelatin it grows very slowly, probably owing in part to the low temperature at which gelatin cultures must be kept. If development occurs it appears as very small whitish or blue-white points on the plates. These very small colonies are round, finely granular, sharply circumscribed, and slightly elevated above the surface of the gelatin. The growth is very slow and no liquefaction of the gelatin occurs.

If grown in slant or stab cultures, the surface development is very limited; along the needle track very small, whitish granules appear. This organism is conspicuous for the rapidity with which it loses its pathogenic properties and the fact that after a very few generations it can no longer be caused to grow.

On agar-agar the colonies are almost transparent; they are more or less glistening and very delicate in their structure.

On blood-serum the growth is more marked, though still extremely feeble. Here it appears as a very delicate film, consisting of fine points growing closely side by side.

A growth on potato has not been observed.

The organism is not motile.

It grows best at a temperature between 35° C.–38° C.

Under 24° C. no growth has been observed, and from 42° C. on, the development is checked.

Under most favorable conditions the growth is very slow. It grows as well without as with oxygen. It is, therefore, one of the facultative anaërobic forms.

The most successful efforts at the cultivation of this organism are those seen when the agar-gelatin mixture of Guarniari is employed. (See this medium.)

It may be stained with the ordinary aniline staining reagents. For demonstration of the capsule the method of Gram gives the best results. (See Stainings.)

b. SEPTICÆMIA OF THE MICROCOCCUS TETRAGENUS.

Should the death of the animal not occur within the first twenty-eight to thirty hours after inoculation, but be postponed until between the fourth and the eighth day, it may occur as a result of invasion of the tissues by the organism now to be described, viz., the micrococcus tetragenus.

This organism was discovered by Gaffky and was subsequently described by Koch in the account of his experiments upon tuberculosis. It is often present in the saliva of healthy individuals and is commonly present in the sputum of tuberculous patients. Koch found it very frequently in the lung cavities of phthisical patients. It, however, plays no part in the etiology of tuberculosis.

It is a small round coccus of about 1 μ transverse diameter. It is seen as single cells, joined in pairs and in threes, but its most conspicuous grouping is in fours, from which arrangement it takes its name. In preparations made from cultures of this organism it is not rare to find here and there single bodies which are much larger than the other individuals in the field. Close inspection reveals these bodies to be cells in the initial stage of division into twos and fours. A peculiarity of this organism is that the cells are seen to be bound together by a transparent gelatinous substance.

When cultivated artificially it grows very slowly.

Upon gelatin plates the colonies appear as round, sharply circumscribed, punctiform masses which are slightly elevated above the surface of the surrounding medium. Under a low magnifying power they are seen to be slightly granular and present a more or less glassy lustre.

The colonies increase but little in size after the third or fourth day. If cultivated as stab cultures in gelatin there appears upon the surface at the point of inoculation a circumscribed white point, slightly elevated above the surface and limited to the immediate neighborhood of the point of inoculation. Down the needle-track the growth is not continuous, but appears in isolated, round, dense white clumps or beads, which do not develop beyond the size of very small points.

It does not liquefy gelatin.

Upon plates of nutrient agar-agar the colonies appear as small, almost transparent, round points, which have about the same color as a drop of egg-albumin; they are very slightly opaque. They are moist and glistening. They rarely develop to an extent exceeding 1 to 2 mm. in diameter.

Upon agar-agar as stab or slant cultures, the surface growth has more or less of a mucoid appearance. It is moist, glistening, and irregularly outlined. The outline of the growth depends upon the moisture of the agar. It is slightly elevated above the surface of the medium.

In contradistinction to the gelatin stab-cultures, the growth is continuous along the track of the needle in the stab cultures upon agar-agar.

The growth on potato is a thick, irregular, slimy-looking patch.

The presence of the transparent gelatinous substance which is seen to surround these organisms renders them coherent, so that efforts to take up a portion of a colony from the agar-agar or potato cultures results usually in drawing out fine silky threads consisting of organisms imbedded in this gelatinous material.

The organism grows best at from 35° C. to 38° C., but can be cultivated at the ordinary room temperature —about 20° C.

The growth under all conditions is not rapid.

It grows both in the presence of and without oxygen. It is not motile.

It stains readily with all the ordinary aniline dyes. In tissues its presence is readily demonstrated by the staining method of Gram.

The grouping into fours is particularly well seen in sections from the organs of animals dead of this form of septicæmia.

In such sections the organisms will always be found within the capillaries.

To the naked eye no alteration can be seen in the organs of animals which have died as a result of inoculation with the micrococcus tetragenus; but microscopic examination of cover-slip preparations from the blood and viscera reveals the presence of the organisms throughout the body—especially is this true of preparations from the spleen. White mice and guinea-pigs are susceptible to the disease. Gray mice, dogs, and rabbits are not susceptible to this form of septicæmia. Subsequent inoculation of healthy animals with a drop of blood, a bit of tissue, or a portion of a pure culture of this organism from the body of an animal dead of the disease, results in a reproduction of the conditions found in the dead animal from which the tissues or cultures were obtained.

It sometimes occurs that in guinea-pigs which have been inoculated with this organism, there results local pus-formations instead of a general septicæmia. The organisms will then be found in the pus-cavity.

CHAPTER XX.

Tuberculosis—Microscopic appearance of miliary tubercles—Encapsulation of tuberculous foci—Diffuse caseation—Cavity-formation—Primary infection—Modes of infection—Location of the bacilli in the tissues—Staining peculiarities.

SHOULD the animal succumb to neither of the septic processes just described, then its death from tuberculosis may be reasonably expected.

When this process is in progress, alterations in the lymphatic glands nearest the seat of inoculation may be detected by the touch in from two to four weeks. They will then be found to be enlarged. Though not constant, tumefaction and subsequent ulceration at the point of inoculation may sometimes be observed. Progressive emaciation, loss of appetite, and difficulty in respiration point to the existence of the tubercular process. Death ensues in from four to eight weeks after inoculation. At autopsy either general or local tuberculosis may be found. The expressions of the tubercular process are so manifold and in different animals differ so widely the one from the other, that no rigid law as to what will be found at autopsy can *à priori* be laid down.

The guinea-pig, which is best suited for this experiment, because of the greater regularity of its susceptibility to the disease over that of other animals usually found in the laboratory, presents, in the main, changes which are characterized by a condition of coagulation, necrosis, and caseation. This is particularly the case when the infection is general, *i. e.*, when the process is of the acute miliary type. This pathological-anatomical alteration is best seen in the tissue of the liver and spleen of these animals, where the condition is most pronounced.

In general, the tubercular lesions can be divided into those of strictly focal character—the miliary and the conglomerate tubercles, and those which are more diffuse in their nature. The latter lesions, although of the same fundamental nature as the miliary tubercles, are much greater in extent and not so sharply circumscribed.

These latter lesions play a greater rôle in the pathology of the disease than do the miliary nodules, although it is to the presence of the latter that the disease owes its name.

At autopsy the pathological manifestations of the disease are not infrequently confined to the seat of inoculation and the neighboring lymphatic glands. These tissues will then present all the characteristics of the tuberculous process in the stage of cheesy degeneration. When the disease is general the degree of its extension varies. Sometimes the small gray nodules—the miliary tubercles—are only to be seen with the naked eye in the tissues of the liver and spleen. Again, they may invade the lungs, and commonly they are distributed over the serous membranes of the intestines, the lungs, the heart, and the brain. These simple gray nodules, as seen by the naked eye, vary in size from that of a pin-point to that of a hempseed, and as a rule are, in this stage, the result of the fusion between two or more smaller miliary foci. Though the two terms, "miliary" and "conglomerate," exist for the description of the macroscopic appearance of these nodules, yet it is very rare that any condition other than that due to the fusion together of several of these minute foci can be detected by the naked eye.

The miliary tubercles are of a pale gray color, with a white centre, are slightly elevated above the surface of the tissue in which they exist, and, as stated, vary considerably in dimensions, usually appearing as points which range in size from that of a pin-point to that of a pin-head. They are not only located upon the surface of the organs, but are distributed through the depths of the tissues. To the touch they sometimes present nothing characteristic, but may frequently, when closely packed together in large numbers, give a mealy or sandy sensation to the fingers. Stained sections of these miliary tubercles present an entirely characteristic appearance, and the disease may be diagnosticated by these histological changes alone, though the crucial test in the diagnosis is the finding of tubercle bacilli in these nodules.

MICROSCOPIC APPEARANCE OF MILIARY TUBERCLES.—The simple miliary tubercles under the low magnifying power of the microscope present somewhat the following appearance: There is a central pale area, evidently composed of necrotic tissue because of its incapacity for taking up the staining employed. Scattered here and there through this necrotic area may be seen granular masses irregular in size and shape. They take up the stains employed and are evidently the fragments of cell-nuclei in the course of destruction. Through the necrotic area may here and there be seen irregular lines, bands, or ridges, the remains of tissues not yet completely destroyed by the necrotic process. Around the periphery of this area may sometimes be noticed large multi-nucleated cells, the nuclei of which are arranged about the periphery of the cell or grouped irregularly at its poles. The arrangement of these nuclei appears in the sections sometimes as ovals, again they are somewhat crescentic in their grouping. In the tubercles from the human subject these large "giant-cells," as they are called, are quite common. They are much less frequent in the tubercular tissues from the lower animals.

Round about this central focus of necrosis is seen a more or less broad zone of closely packed small round and oval bodies which stain readily but not homogeneously. They vary in size and shape, and are seen to be imbedded in a delicate network of fibrous-looking tissue.

This fibrous-looking network in which these bodies lie, and which is a common accompaniment of giant-cell formation, is in part composed of fibrin, but is in the main most probably the remains of the interstitial fibrous tissue of the part. This zone of which we are speaking, is the zone of so-called "granulation tissue," and consists of leucocytes, granulation cells, and the fibrous remains of the part; the irregularly oval, granular bodies which take up the staining are the nuclei of these cells. The zone of granulation tissue surrounds the whole of the tubercular process, and at its periphery fades gradually into the healthy surrounding tissue or fuses with a similar zone surrounding another tubercular focus. This may be taken as the description of a typical miliary tubercle.

DIFFUSE CASEATION.—The diffuse caseation, as said, plays a more important rôle in the tuberculous lesion, both in the human and experimental forms, than does the formation of miliary tubercles. In this a large area of tissue undergoes the same process of necrosis and caseation as the centre of the miliary tubercle. In some tissues it is more marked than in others. These tissues are the lungs and the lymph-glands. In rabbits, particularly, all the changes in the lung frequently come under this head. When this is the case solid masses are found, sometimes as large as a pea, or involving even an entire lobe or the whole lung in some cases. They are of a whitish-yellow, opaque color, and on section are peculiarly dry and hard. Entire lymphatic glands may be changed in this way. The conditions for this caseation of the tissues are probably given when a large number of tubercle bacilli enter the tissue simultaneously and a wide area is involved, instead of the small centre of the miliary tubercle. Necrosis is so rapid that time is not given for those reactive changes to take place in the tissues which result in the formation of the outer zone of the miliary tubercle. In other instances the entire caseous area is surrounded by a zone similar to that around the caseous centre of the miliary tubercles. It is of special importance to recognize the connection between this diffuse caseation of the tissue and the tubercle bacilli, because until its nature was accurately determined the caseous pneumonia of the lungs formed the chief obstacle which many had in recognizing the infectiousness of tuberculosis.

CAVITY-FORMATION.—The production of cavities which forms such a prominent feature in human tuberculosis, particularly in the lungs, is due to the softening of the necrotic caseous masses or of aggregations of miliary tubercles. The material softens and is expelled, and a cavity remains. In the wall of this cavity the tuberculous changes still proceed, both as a diffuse caseation and formation of miliary tubercles. The whole cavity with the reactive changes in the tissues of its walls may be considered as representing a single tubercle, its wall forming a tissue very analogous to the outer zone of the single tubercle, the cavity itself corresponding to the caseous centre. In the lower animals cavity-formation of this sort is very rare, owing to the greater resistance of the caseous tissue.

In the contents and in the walls of tubercular cavities bacteria other than the tubercle bacilli are found. It is to the influence of some of these, as we have just seen, that diseases other than tuberculosis may sometimes be produced by the inoculation of lower animals with the sputum from such cases.

ENCAPSULATION OF TUBERCULAR FOCI.—It not uncommonly occurs that round about a necrotic tubercular focus there is formed a fibrous capsule which may completely cut off the diseased from the healthy tissue surrounding it. Or a tubercular focus may, through the resistance of the tissue in which it is located, be more or less completely isolated. In this condition the diseased foci may lie dormant for a long time and give no evidence of their existence, until by some intercurrent interference they are caused to break through their envelopes. With the passage of the bacilli or their spores from the central foci into the vascular or lymphatic circulation the disease may then become general.

It is to some such accident as this that the sudden appearance of general tubercular infection in subjects supposed to have recovered from the primary local manifestations may often be attributed. The breaking-down of old caseous lymphatic glands is a common example of this condition.

PRIMARY INFECTION.—The primary infection occurs through either the vascular or lymphatic circulation·

Through these channels the bacilli gain access to the tissues and become lodged in the finer capillary ramifications or in the more minute lymph-spaces. Here they find conditions favorable to their development, and in the course of this process produce substances of a chemical nature which act directly in bringing about the death of the tissues in their immediate neighborhood. This tissue-death is probably the very first effect of the bacilli in the body, and represents the necrotic centre, which can always be seen in even the most minute tubercles. With the production of this progressive necrosis—for progressive it is, as it continues as long as the bacilli live and continue to produce their poisonous products—there is in addition a reactive change in the surrounding tissues which consists in the formation of the granulation zone at the outer margins of the dying and dead tissue. This zone consists of small, round granulation-cells and of leucocytes, all of which are seen in the meshes of the finer fibrous tissues of the part. At the same time alterations are produced in the walls of the vessels going to the part; this tends to occlude them, and thus the process of tissue-death is favored by a diminution of the amount of nutrition brought to them. These changes continue until eventually the life processes of the bacilli are checked, or conglomerate tubercles, widespread caseation, or cavity-formation results.

MODES OF INFECTION.—Experimentally, tuberculosis may be produced in susceptible animals by subcutaneous inoculation, by direct injection into the circulation, by injection into the peritoneal cavity, by feeding of tuberculous material, and by the introduction of the bacilli into the air-passages.

In the human subject the most common portals of infection are doubtless the air-passages, the alimentary tract, and cutaneous wounds. When introduced subcutaneously the resulting process finds its most pronounced expression in the lymphatic system. The growing bacilli make their way into the fine lymphatic spaces of the loose cellular tissue, are taken up in the lymph stream and deposited in the neighboring lymphatic glands. Here they may remain, and give rise to no alteration further than that seen in the glands themselves, or they may pass on to neighboring glands and eventually be disseminated throughout the whole lymphatic system, ultimately reaching the vascular system.

When having gained access to the bloodvessels, the results are the same as those following upon intravascular injection of the bacilli: general tuberculosis quickly follows, with the most conspicuous production of miliary tubercles in the lungs and kidneys, less numerous in the spleen, liver, and bone marrow.

When inhaled into the lungs, if conditions are favorable, multiplication of the bacilli quickly follows. With their growth they are mechanically pressed into the tissues of the lungs; as multiplication continues some are transported from the primary seat of infection to healthy portions of the lung tissue, there to give rise to a further production of the tubercular process.

In the same way infection through the alimentary tract is in the main due to the mechanical pressure of the bacilli upon the walls of the intestines. Investigation has shown that lesions of the intestinal coats are not necessary for the entrance of the tubercle bacilli from the intestines into the body. They may be transported from the intestinal tract into the lymphatics in the same way that the fat droplets of the chyle find entrance into the lymphatic circulation.

The evidence produced by Cornet points to the lungs as the most common portals of natural infection for the human being. Unlike most pathogenic organisms, the tubercle bacillus has the property of forming spores within the tissues. These spores, which are highly resistant and are not destroyed by drying, are thrown off from the lungs in the sputum of tuberculous patients in large number, and unless special precautions are taken to prevent it the sputum becomes dried, is ground into dust and sets free in the atmosphere the spores of tubercle bacilli which came with it from the lungs. The frequency of pulmonary tuberculosis points to this as one of the commonest sources of infection.

LOCATION OF THE BACILLI IN THE TISSUES.—The bacilli will be found to be most numerous in those tissues which are in the active stage of the process.

In the very initial stage of the disease the bacilli will be fewer in number than later. At this stage only here and there single rods may be found; later they will be more numerous, and finally, when the process has advanced to a stage easily recognizable by the naked eye, they will be found in the granulation zones in clumps and scattered about in large numbers.

In the central necrotic masses, which consist of cell detritus, it is rare that the organisms can be demonstrated microscopically. It is at the periphery of these areas and in the progressing granular zone that they are most frequently to be seen.

This apparent absence of the bacilli from the central necrotic area must not be taken, however, as evidence that this tissue does not contain them. As bacilli, they are difficult to demonstrate here because the probabilities are that in this locality, owing to conditions unfavorable to their further growth, they are in the spore stage, a stage in which it is as yet impossible, with our present methods of staining, to render them visible. The fact that this tissue is infective, and with it the disease can be reproduced in susceptible animals, speaks for the accuracy of this assumption. A conspicuous example of this condition is seen in old scrofulous glands. These glands present usually a slow process, are commonly caseous, and always possess the property of producing the disease when introduced into the tissues of susceptible animals, and yet they are the most difficult of all tissues in which to demonstrate microscopically the presence of tubercle bacilli. In tubercles containing giant-cells the bacilli can usually be demonstrated in the granular contents of these cells. Frequently, they will be found accumulated at the pole of the cell opposite to that occupied by the nuclei, as if there existed an antagonism between the nuclei and the bacilli. In some of these cells, however, the distribution of the bacilli is seen to be irregular and they will be found scattered among the nuclei as well as in the necrotic centre of the cell.

As the number of bacilli in the giant-cell increases the cell itself is ultimately destroyed.

Tubercular tissues always contain the bacilli or their spores and are always capable of reproducing the disease when introduced into the body of a susceptible animal. From the tissues of this animal the bacilli may again be obtained and cultivated artificially, and these cultures are capable of again producing the disease when further inoculated. Thus the postulates which are necessary to prove the etiological rôle of the organism in the production of this malady are all fulfilled.

THE TUBERCLE BACILLUS.—Of the three pathogenic organisms of which we are speaking, the tubercle bacillus will give us most difficulty in our efforts at cultivation.

It is in the strict sense of the word a parasite and finds conditions entirely favorable to its development only in the animal body. On ordinary artificial media the bacilli taken directly from the animal body grow only very imperfectly or in many cases not at all. From this it seems probable that there is a difference in the nature of the individual bacilli of this group—some appearing to be capable only of growth in the animal tissues, while others are apparently possessed of the power to lead a limited saprophytic existence. It may be, therefore, that those bacilli which we obtain as artificial cultures from the animal body are offsprings from the more saprophytic members of the group. At best, one never sees with the tubercle bacillus a saprophytic condition in any way comparable to that possessed by many of the other organisms with which we have to deal.

In efforts to cultivate this organism directly from the tissues of the animal, the method by which one obtains the best results is that recommended by Koch—cultivation upon blood-serum. So strictly is this organism a parasite that very limited alterations in the conditions under which it is growing may result in failure to successfully study it. It is, therefore, necessary that the injunctions for obtaining it in pure culture should be carefully observed.

The blood-serum upon which the organism is to be cultivated should be comparatively freshly prepared—that is, it should not be dry.

PREPARATION OF CULTURES FROM TISSUES.— Under strictest antiseptic precautions, remove from the animal the tubercular tissue—the liver, spleen, or a lymphatic gland being preferable. Place the tissue in a sterilized Petri dish and dissect out with sterilized scissors and forceps the small tubercular nodules. Place each nodule upon the surface of the blood-serum, one nodule in each tube, and with a heavy, sterilized, looped platinum needle or spatula, rub it carefully over the surface of the blood-serum. It is best to dissect away twenty to thirty such tubercles and treat each in the same way. Some of the tubes will remain sterile, others may be contaminated by outside organisms during the manipulation, while a few may give the result desired—a growth of the bacilli themselves.

After inoculating the tubes they should be carefully sealed up to prevent evaporation and consequent drying. This is best done by burning off the superfluous overhanging cotton plug in the gas-flame, and then impregnating the upper layers of the cotton with either sealing-wax or paraffin of a high melting-point. This precaution is necessary because of the slow growth of the organism. Under the most favorable conditions tubercle bacilli directly from the animal body show no evidence of growth for about twelve days after inoculation upon blood-serum, and, as they must be retained during this time at the body temperature— 37.5° C.—evaporation would take place very rapidly and the medium become too dry for their development.

If these primary efforts result in the appearance of a culture of the bacilli, further cultivations may be made by taking up a bit of the colony, preferably a moderately large quantity, and transferring it to fresh serum, and this in turn is sealed up and retained at the same temperature. Once having obtained the organism in pure culture its subsequent cultivation may be conducted upon the glycerin-agar-agar mixture—ordinary neutral nutrient agar-agar to which 6 or 7 per cent. of glycerin has been added. This is a very favorable medium for the growth of this organism after once having established its saprophytic form of existence, though blood-serum is perhaps the best medium to be employed in obtaining the first generation of the organism from the tubercular tissues.

The organism may be cultivated also on neutral milk to which 1 per cent. of agar-agar has been added, also upon the surface of potato, and likewise in meat infusion bouillon to which 6 or 7 per cent. of glycerin has been added.

In appearance the cultures of the tubercle bacilli are characteristic—after once having seen them there is but little probability of subsequent mistake.

They appear as dry masses, which may develop upon the surface of the medium either as flat scales or as clumps of mealy-looking granules. They are never moist, and frequently have the appearance of coarse meal which had been spread upon the surface of the medium. In the lower part of the tube in which they are growing (that part occupied by a few drops of fluid which has in part been squeezed from the medium during the process of solidification, and is in part water of condensation) the colonies may be seen to float as a thin pellicle upon the surface.

The individuals making up the growth adhere so tenaciously together that it is with the greatest difficulty that they can be completely separated. In even the oldest and dryest cultures pulverization is impossible. The masses can only be separated and broken up by grinding in a mortar with the addition of some foreign substance, such as very fine, sterilized sand, dust, etc.

The cultures are of a dirty-drab or brownish-gray color when seen on serum or on glycerin-agar-agar.

On potato they grow in practically the same way, though the development is much more limited. They are here of nearly the same color as the potato on which they are growing.

On milk-agar-agar they are of so nearly the same color as the medium, that unless they are growing as the mealy-looking masses considerably elevated above the surface, their presence is less conspicuous than when on the other media.

In bouillon they appear as a thin pellicle on the surface. This may fall to the bottom of the fluid and continue to develop, its place on the surface being taken by a second pellicle.

Under all conditions of artificial development the cultures of this organism are always very dry and brittle in appearance, though in truth the individuals adhere tenaciously together by a very glutinous substance.

The tubercle bacillus does not develop on gelatin, because of the low temperature at which this medium must be used.

MICROSCOPIC APPEARANCE OF THE TUBERCLE BACILLUS.—Microscopically the organism itself is a delicate rod, usually somewhat beaded in its structure, though rarely it is seen to be homogeneous. It is either quite straight or somewhat curved or bent on its long axis. In some preparations involution-forms, consisting of rods a little clubbed at one extremity or slightly bulging at different points, may be detected. It varies in length—sometimes being seen in very short segments, again much longer. On an average its length is seen to vary from 2 to 5 μ. It is commonly described as being in length about one-fourth to one-half the diameter of a red blood-corpuscle. It is very slender.

These rods usually present, as has been said, an appearance of alternate stained and colorless portions. It is the latter portions which are believed to be the spores of the organism, though as yet no absolute proof of this opinion has been established.

At times these colorless portions are seen to bulge slightly beyond the contour of the rod, and in this way give to the rods the beaded appearance so commonly ascribed to them.

STAINING PECULIARITIES.—A peculiarity of this organism is its behavior toward staining reagents, and by this means alone it may be easily recognized. The tubercle bacilli do not stain by the ordinary methods. They possess some peculiarity in their composition which renders them more or less proof against the simpler dyes. It is therefore necessary that more energetic and penetrating reagents than the ordinary watery solutions should be employed Experience has taught us that certain substances not only increase the solubility of the aniline coloring substances, but by their presence the penetration of the coloring agents is very much increased. These substances are aniline oil and carbolic acid. They are both present in the point of the solutions to about saturation. (For the exact proportions see chapter on Staining Reagents.)

Under the influence of heat, these solutions are seen

to stain all bacteria very intensely—the tubercle bacilli as well as the ordinary forms. If we subject our preparation, which may contain a mixture of tubercle bacilli and other forms, to the action of decolorizing agents, another peculiarity of the tubercle bacilli will be observed. While all other organisms in the preparation will give up their color and become invisible, the tubercle bacilli retain it with marked tenacity. They stain with great difficulty, but once stained they retain the color even under the influence of strong decolorizing agents.

The only other organism possessing a similar peculiarity is the bacillus of leprosy, with which, under ordinary conditions, we are not likely to come in contact. This micro-chemical reaction therefore serves as a means of differentiating this organism in sputum and other fluids from the body of suspected subjects from all other bacteria that are likely to be present.

SUSCEPTIBILITY OF ANIMALS TO TUBERCULOSIS.—The animals which are known to be susceptible to the tubercular processes are man, apes, cattle, horses, sheep, guinea-pigs, pigeons, rabbits, cats, and field mice.

White mice, dogs, and rats possess immunity against the disease.

We have reviewed the three common pathogenic organisms with which we may come in contact in the sputum of tuberculous individuals. Occasionally other forms may be present. The pyogenic forms are not rarely found, and for a long time after diphtheria the bacillus of Löffler is known to be demonstrable in the pharynx. These latter organisms will be described under their proper heads.

CHAPTER XXI.

Suppuration—The staphylococcus pyogenes aureus.

PREPARE from the pus of an acute abscess or boil, which has been opened under antiseptic precautions, a set of plates of agar-agar. Care must be given that none of the antiseptic fluid gains access to the culture tubes, otherwise its antiseptic effect may be seen and the development of the organisms interfered with. It is best, therefore, to take up a drop of the pus upon the platinum-wire loop after it has been flowing for a few seconds; even then it must be taken from the mouth of the wound and before it has run over the surface of the skin. At the same time prepare two or three cover-slips from the pus.

Microscopic examination of these slips will reveal the presence of a large number of pus-cells, both multi-nucleated and with horseshoe-shaped nuclei, some threads of disintegrated connective-tissue, and, lying here and there throughout the preparation, small round bodies which will sometimes appear singly, sometimes in pairs, and frequently will be seen grouped together somewhat after the manner of clusters of grapes. They stain readily and are commonly located in the material between the pus-cells; *very rarely* they may be seen in the protoplasmic body of the cell. (Compare the preparation with a similar one made from the pus of gonorrhœa. In what way do the two preparations differ the one from the other?)

After twenty-four hours in the incubator the plates will be seen to be studded here and there with yellow or orange-colored colonies, which are usually round, moist, and glistening in their naked-eye appearances. Under the low-power hand-lens they are frequently irregularly star-shaped or lobulated in outline and appear very dense in structure. Under the low objective they appear, when on the surface, as coarsely granular, irregularly round patches, with more or less ragged borders and a dark irregular central mass, which has somewhat the appearance of masses of coarser clumps of the same material as that composing the rest of the colony. When deep down in the culture medium they present but little that is typical. Microscopically, these colonies are composed of small round cells, irregularly grouped together. They are in every way of the same appearance as those seen upon the cover-slip preparations.

Prepare from one of these colonies a pure stab culture in gelatin. After thirty-six to forty-eight hours liquefaction of the gelatin along the track of the needle, and most conspicuous at its upper end, will be observed. As growth continues the liquefaction becomes more or less of a stocking-shape, and gradually widens out at its upper end into an irregular funnel. This will continue until the whole of the gelatin in the tube eventually becomes fluid. There can always be noticed at the bottom of the liquefying portion an orange-colored or yellow mass composed of a number of the organisms which have sunk to the bottom of the fluid.

On potato the growth is quite luxuriant, appearing as a brilliant orange-colored layer, somewhat lobulated and a little less moist then when growing upon agar. It does not produce fermentation with gas-production. It belongs to the group of facultative aërobes.

In milk it rapidly brings about coagulation with acid reaction.

It is not motile, and being of the family of micrococci, does not form endogenous spores. It possesses, however, a marked resistance toward detrimental agencies.

In bouillon it causes a diffuse clouding, and after a time presents a yellow sedimentation.

This organism is the commonest of the pathogenic bacteria with which we shall meet. It is the staphylococcus pyogenes aureus, and is the organism most frequently concerned in the production of acute, circumscribed, suppurative inflammations. It is almost everywhere present, and is the organism most dreaded by the surgeon.

In studying its effects upon lower animals a number of points are to be remembered. While it is the etiological factor in the production of most of the suppurative processes in man, still it is with no little difficulty that these conditions can be reproduced in the lower animals. Its subcutaneous introduction into their tissues does not always result in abscess-formation, and when it does there seems to have been some coincident interference with the circulation in these tissues which render them less able to resist its inroads. When introduced into the great serous cavities of the lower animals it is not always followed by the production of inflammation. If the abdominal cavity of a dog, for example, be carefully opened so as to make as slight a wound as possible, and no injury be done to the intestines, large quantities of bouillon cultures or watery suspensions of this organism may, and repeatedly have been introduced into the peritoneum without the slightest injury to the animal. On the contrary, if some substance which acts as a direct irritant to the intestines —such, for example, as a small bit of potato upon which the organisms are growing—is at the same time introduced, or the intestines be mechanically injured, so that there is a disturbance in their circulation, then the introduction of these organisms is promptly followed by acute and fatal peritonitis.

On the other hand, the results which follow their introduction into the circulation are practically constant. If one injects into the circulation of the rabbit through one of the veins of the ear, or in any other way, from 0.1 to 0.3 c.c. of a bouillon culture or watery suspension of this organism, a fatal pyæmia always follows in from two and one-half to three days. A few hours before death the animal is frequently seen to have severe convulsions. Now and then excessive secretion of urine is noticed. The animal may appear in moderately good condition until from eight to ten hours before death. At the autopsy a typical picture presents. The voluntary muscles are seen to be marked here and there by yellow spots, which average the size of a flax-seed, and are of about the same shape. They lie usually with their long axis running longitudinally between the muscle fibres. As the abdominal and thoracic cavities are opened the diaphragm is not rarely seen to be studded by them. Frequently the pericardial sac is distended with a clear gelatinous fluid, and almost constantly the yellow points are to be seen in the myocardium. The kidneys are rarely without them; here they appear on the surface scattered about as single yellow points, or again, are seen as conglomerate masses of small yellow points which occupy, as a rule, the area fed by a single vessel. If one makes a section into one of these yellow points it will be seen to extend deep down through the substance of the kidney as a yellow, wedge-shaped mass, the base of the wedge being at the surface of the organ.

It is very rare that these abscesses—for abscesses these yellow points are, as we shall see when we come to study them more closely—are found either in the liver, spleen, or brain; their usual location being, as said, in the kidney, myocardium, and voluntary muscles.

These minute abscesses contain a dry, cheesy, necrotic centre, in which the staphylococci are present in large numbers, as may be seen upon cover-slips prepared from them. They may also be obtained in pure culture from these suppurating points.

Preserve in Müller's fluid and in alcohol duplicate bits of all the tissue in which the abscesses are located.

When these tissues are hard enough to cut, sections should be made through the abscess-points, and the histological changes carefully studied.

MICROSCOPIC STUDY OF COVER-SLIPS AND SECTIONS. —In cover-slip preparations this organism stains readily with the ordinary dyes.

In tissues, however, it is best to employ some method by means of which contrast stains may be employed, and the location and grouping of the organisms in the tissues rendered more conspicuous.

When stained, sections of tissues containing these small abscesses present the following appearances:

To the naked eye will be seen here and there in the section, if the abscesses are very numerous, small, darkly stained areas which range in size from that of a pin-point up to those having a diameter of from 1 to 2 mm.

These points, when in the kidney, may be round or oval in outline, or may appear wedge-shaped, with the base of the wedge toward the surface of the organ. The differences in shape depend frequently upon the direction in which the section has been made through the kidney. In the muscles they are irregularly round or oval.

When quite small they appear to the naked eye as simple, round or oval, darkly stained points, but when they are more advanced a pale centre can usually be made out.

When magnified, they appear in the earliest stages as minute aggregations of small cells, the nuclei of which stain intensely. Almost always there can be seen about the centre of these cell-accumulations evidences of progressing necrosis. The normal structure of the cells of the tissue will be more or less destroyed; there will be seen a granular condition due to cell-fragmentation; at different points about the centre of this area the tissue will appear cloudy and the tissue-cells will not stain readily. All about and through this spot will be seen the nuclei of pus cells, many of which are undergoing disintegration. In the smallest of these beginning abscesses the staphylococci are to be seen scattered here and there about the centre of the necrotic tissue, but in a more advanced stage they are commonly seen massed together in very large numbers in the form commonly referred to as *emboli of micrococci*.

The localized necrosis of the tissues which is seen at the centre of the abscess is the direct result of the action of a poison produced by the bacteria, and is the starting-point for all abscess-formations.

When the process is somewhat advanced the different parts of the abscess are more easily detected. They then present in sections somewhat the following conditions:

At the centre can be seen a dense, granular mass, which stains readily with the aniline dyes and, when highly magnified, is found to be made up of staphylococci. Sometimes the shape of this mass of staphylococci corresponds to that of the capillary in which the organisms became lodged and developed. Immediately about the embolus of cocci the tissues are seen to be in an advanced stage of necrosis. Their structure is almost completely destroyed, though it is seen to be more advanced in some of the elements of the tissues than in others. As we approach the periphery of this faintly stained necrotic area, it becomes marked here and there with granular bodies, irregular in size and shape, which stain in the same way as do the nuclei of the pus-cells and represent the result of disintregation going on in these cells.

Beyond this we come upon a dense, deeply stained zone, consisting of closely packed pus-cells; of granular detritus resulting from destructive processes acting upon these cells; and of the normal cellular and connective-tissue elements of the part. Here and there through this zone will be seen localized areas of beginning death of the tissues. This zone gradually fades away into the healthy surrounding tissues. It constitutes the so-called "abscess wall."

Such is the picture presented by the miliary abscess when produced experimentally in the rabbit, and it corresponds throughout with the pathological changes which accompany the formation of larger abscesses in the tissues of human beings.

From these small abscesses in the tissues of the rabbit the staphylococcus pyogenes aureus may again be obtained in pure culture, and will present identically the same characteristics that were possessed by the culture with which the animal was inoculated.

THE LESS COMMON PYOGENIC ORGANISMS.—
The pus of an acute abscess in the human being may
sometimes contain other organisms beside the staphylococcus pyogenes aureus. The staphylococcus pyogenes
albus and citreus may be found. The colonies of the
former are white, those of the latter are lemon-color.
The streptococcus pyogenes is also sometimes present.
The commonest of the pyogenic organisms however is
that just described—the staphylococcus pyogenes aureus.

THE STREPTOCOCCUS PYOGENES.—From a spreading
phlegmonous inflammation prepare cultures. What is
the predominating organism? Does it appear as irregular clusters of grapes, or has its individuals a definite
regular arrangement? Are its colonies like those of the
staphylococcus pyogenes aureus?

Isolate this organism in pure cultures. In these cultures it will be found to present an arrangement somewhat like a chain of beads. Determine its cultural
peculiarities and describe them accurately.

This is the streptococcus pyogenes, and is the organism most commonly found in rapidly *spreading* suppuration in contradistinction to the staphylococcus pyogenes
aureus, which is most frequently found in *circumscribed*
abscess-formations; they may be found together.

If the opportunity presents, obtain cultures from a
case of erysipelas. Compare the organism thus obtained
with the streptococcus just mentioned. Inoculate a rabbit
both subcutaneously and into the circulation with about
0.2 c.c. of a pure bouillon culture of these organisms.
Do the results correspond, and do they in any way
suggest the results obtained with the staphylococcus
pyogenes aureus when introduced into animals in the
same way? Do these streptococci flourish readily on
ordinary media?

CHAPTER XXII.

Typhoid fever—Study of the organism concerned in its production.

THE organism, discovered by Eberth and by Gaffky, which is recognized as the etiological factor in the production of typhoid fever, may be described as follows:

In patients suffering from this disease it has been found during life in the blood, urine, and feces, and at autopies in the tissues of the spleen, liver, kidneys, intestinal lymphatic glands, and intestines.

It is a bacillus about three times as long as it is broad, with rounded ends. It may appear at one time as very short ovals, at another time as long threads. Its breadth remains tolerably constant. Its morphology presents nothing that will aid in its identification. It stains a little less readily with the aniline dyes than do most of the other organisms. It is very actively motile, and when stained by the special method of Löffler (see this method in chapter on Stainings) is seen to possess very delicate locomotive organs in the form of fine, hair-like flagellæ, which are given off in large numbers from all parts of its surface. These flagellæ are not seen in unstained preparations, or are they rendered visible by the ordinary methods of staining.

GELATIN PLATES.—Its growth, when seen in the depths of the medium, has nothing characteristic, appearing simply as round or oval, finely granular points. On the surface it develops as very superficial, blue-white colonies, with irregular borders. They are a little denser at the centre than at the periphery. When magnified, the colonies present wrinkles or folds, which give to them, in miniature, the appearance seen in the relief maps which represent mountainous districts. These colonies have sometimes the appearance of flattened pellicles of glass-wool, and glisten with more or less of a bronze color.

ON AGAR-AGAR the colonies present nothing typical.

STAB CULTURES.—In stab cultures the growth is mostly on the surface, there being only a very limited development down the track made by the needle. The surface growth has the same appearance in general as that given for the colonies.

POTATO.—The growth on potato is usually described as luxuriant but invisible, making its presence evident only by the production of a slight increase of moisture at the inoculated point, and by a limited resistance offered to the needle when scraped across the track of growth.

POTATO GELATIN.—The growth is similar to that upon ordinary nutrient gelatin.

MILK.—It does not cause coagulation when grown in sterilized milk.

It does not liquefy gelatin.

It grows both with and without oxygen.

It does not produce indol.

In bouillon it causes a uniform clouding of the medium and brings about a slightly acid reaction.

It does not grow rapidly.

It does not produce fermentation with liberation of gas.

It does not form spores. The irregularities of staining so commonly seen in this organism have in some instances led to the belief that the pale, unstained portions of the bacilli indicate the presence of spores. More exact tests, however, have demonstrated the error of this opinion.

It grows at any temperature between 20° C. and 38° C., though more favorably at the latter point.

It is very sensitive to high temperatures, being killed by an exposure of ten minutes to 60° C., and in a much shorter time to slightly higher temperatures.

Owing to a tendency toward retraction of its protoplasm from the cell envelope and the consequent production of vacuoles in the bacilli, the staining of this organism is usually more or less irregular. At some points in a single cell marked differences in the intensity of the staining will be seen, and here and there areas quite free from color can commonly be detected.

PRESENCE IN TISSUES.—It is not easy to demonstrate this organism in tissues unless it is present in large numbers. The manipulations to which the sections are subjected in being mounted rob the bacilli of their staining, and render them invisible, or nearly so. If, however, sections be stained in the carbolic-fuchsin solution, either at the ordinary temperature of the room for from eighteen to twenty hours, or at a higher temperature (40° to 45° C.) for a shorter time, then washed out in absolute alcohol, and cleared up in xylol and mounted in balsam, as a rule, the bacilli (particularly if the tissue is the liver or spleen) can readily be detected massed together in their characteristic clumps. If used in the same way, the methylene-blue solution gives also very satisfactory results.

In searching for the typhoid bacilli in tissues, their

mode of growth under these circumstances must always be borne in mind, otherwise much labor will be expended in vain. In tissues the typhoid bacilli do not lie scattered about in the same way as do the organisms in tissues from cases of septicæmia. They are not regularly distributed along the course of the capillaries; they are localized in small clumps through the tissues, and it is for these clumps, which are easily detected under the low-power objective, that one should search. When the section is prepared for examination, if it is gone over with the low-power objective, one will notice here and there little masses that look in every respect like particles of staining-matter which have been precipitated upon the section at that point. If these little masses are examined with a higher power objective, they will be found to consist of small ovals or short rods so closely packed together that the individuals composing the clump can be seen only at the very periphery of the mass. This is the characteristic appearance of the typhoid organism in tissues. The little masses are usually in the neighborhood of a capillary.

RESULT OF INOCULATION INTO LOWER ANIMALS.—A great many experiments have been made with the view of reproducing the pathological conditions of this disease, as seen in man, in the tissues of lower animals, but with limited success. Fatal results without the appearance of the typical pathological changes have frequently followed these attempts, but in most cases they could be easily traced to the toxic,[1] rather than to the

[1] Toxic—poisonous results not necessarily accompanied by the growth of organisms in the tissues.

truly infective[1] action of the materials introduced into the animals.

The most successful efforts for the production of the typical typhoid lesions in lower animals are those recently reported by Cygnæus. By the introduction of the typhoid bacilli into the tissues of dogs, rabbits, and mice he was able to produce in the small intestines conditions which were histologically and to the naked eye analogous to those found in the human subject.

Of a number of experiments made by the writer with the same object in view, only one positive result followed the introduction of typhoid bacilli into the circulation of rabbits. In this case the ulcer in the ileum was macroscopically and microscopically identical with those found at autopsy in the small intestine of the human subject dead of this disease. The typhoid bacilli were not only obtained from the spleen of the animal by culture methods, but were also demonstrated microscopically in their characteristic clumps in sections of the organ.

Because of the variations in the morphology and cultural peculiarities of this organism, and because of the difficulty experienced in efforts to reproduce in lower animals the conditions found in the human subject, typhoid fever is bacteriologically one of the most unsatisfactory of the infectious diseases.

There are a number of other organisms which botanically appear to be so closely related to the typhoid bacillus, and which, with our present methods for studying these organisms, so closely simulate it, that the difficulty

---

[1] Infective or septic—poisoning of the tissues as a result of the growth of bacteria in them.

of identifying this organism is very great. In addition to this, the variability constantly seen in pure cultures of the typhoid bacillus itself in no way renders the task more simple.

For example, the morphology of the typhoid bacillus is conspicuously inconstant; its growth on potato, which is usually given as characteristic, may, with the same culture, at one time appear as the typical invisible development, at another time it may grow in a way easily to be seen with the naked eye; the change of reaction which it is said to produce in bouillon is sometimes much more intense than at others.

The only properties possessed by it that may be said to be constant are its motility, the absence of indol-production, and its growth on gelatin plates; but there are other organisms which possess these same characteristics in a degree that renders their differentiation from the typhoid organism a matter of extreme difficulty, if not of impossibility.

These points should be borne in mind in the examination of drinking-water supposed to be contaminated by typhoid dejections, for the organisms which most nearly approach the typhoid bacillus in growth and morphology are just those organisms which would appear in water contaminated from cesspools, *i. e.*, the organisms constantly found in the normal intestinal tract. Even in the stools of typhoid-fever patients the presence of these normal inhabitants of the intestinal tract renders the isolation of the typhoid organisms no small task.

The spleen of a patient dead of typhoid fever is the safest place from which to obtain cultures of this organism for study. But it must always be remembered that even here the bacterium coli communis, the normal organism of the colon, is not unlikely to be found. This organism, however, always grows visibly on potato, coagulates milk, produces a more pronounced pink color in litmus-milk than does the typhoid bacillus, and is much less actively motile.

Obtain a pure culture of typhoid bacilli and from this make inoculations upon a series of potatoes of different age and from different sources. Do they all grow alike?

Make a series of twelve tubes of peptone solution to which rosolic acid has been added. Inoculate them all with as near the same amount of material as possible (one loopful from a bouillon culture into each tube); place them all in the incubator. Is the color-change, as compared with the control tube, the same in all cases?

Compare the morphology of cultures of the same age on gelatin, agar-agar, and potato.

Select a culture in which the vacuolations are quite marked. Examine this culture unstained. Do the organisms look as if they contained spores? How would you demonstrate that the vacuolations are not spores?

Obtain from the normal feces a pure culture of the commonest organism present. Write a full description of it. Now make parallel cultures of this organism and of the typhoid organism on all the different media. How do they differ? In what respects are they similar?

CHAPTER XXIII.

Study of the bacillus of anthrax, and the effects produced by its inoculation into animals — Peculiarities of the organism under varying conditions of surroundings.

THE discovery that the blood of animals suffering from splenic fever, or anthrax, always contained minute rod shaped bodies (Pollender, 1855; Davaine, 1863), led to a closer study of this disease, and has resulted, probably, in contributing more to our knowledge of bacteriology in general than work upon any of the other infectious maladies.

The outcome of these investigations is that a rod-shaped microörganism, now known as the bacillus of anthrax, is always present in the blood of animals suffering from this disease; that this organism can be obtained from the tissues of these animals in pure cultures, and that these artificial cultures of the bacillus of anthrax when introduced into the body of susceptible animals can again produce a condition identical to that found in the animal from which they were obtained.

The disease is a true septicæmia, and the capillaries throughout the body after death will always be found to contain the typical rod-shaped organism in larger or smaller numbers.

This organism, when isolated in pure cultures, is seen to be a bacillus which varies considerably in its length, ranging from short rods of 2 to 3 μ in length to longer rods of 20 to 25 μ in length. In breadth it is from 1 to 1.25 μ. Frequently very long threads made up of several rods, joined end to end, are seen.

As it is obtained from the body of the animal, it is usually in the form of short rods *square at the ends.*

When cultivated artificially at the temperature of the body, the bacillus of anthrax presents a series of very interesting stages.

The short rods develop into long threads, which may be seen twisted or plaited together after the manner of ropes, each thread being marked by the points of junction of the short rods composing it.

In this condition it remains until alterations in its surroundings, most conspicuously diminution in its nutritive supply, favor the production of spores. When this stage begins, alterations in the protoplasm of the bacilli may be noticed; they become marked by irregular, granular bodies, which eventually coalesce into glistening, oval spores, one of which lies in nearly every segment of the long thread, and gives to the thread the appearance of a string of glistening beads. In this stage they remain but a short time. The chains of spores, which are held together by the remains of the cells in which they formed, become broken up, and eventually nothing but free oval spores, and here and there the remains of mature bacilli which have undergone degenerative changes, can be found. In this condition the spores, capable of resisting deleterious influences, remain and, unless their surroundings are altered, have been seen to continue in this living, though inactive, condition for a very long time. When placed under favorable conditions again, each spore will germinate into a mature cell, and the same series of changes will be repeated until the favorable surroundings become again gradually unfavorable to development, when the spore-formation is again seen. The spore-formation takes place only at temperatures ranging from 18° to 43° C., 37.50° C. being the most favorable temperature. Under 12° C. they are not formed. With this organism, spore-formation does not occur in the tissues of the living animal, its usual condition at this time being that of short rods. Occasionally, however, somewhat longer forms may be seen.

The bacillus of anthrax is not motile.

GROWTH ON AGAR-AGAR.—The colonies of this organism, as seen upon agar-agar, present a very typical appearance, from which they have been likened unto the hair of a Medusa. From a central point which is more or less dense, consisting of a felt-like mass of long threads matted irregularly together, the growth continues outward upon the surface of the agar. It is made up of wavy bundles in which the threads are seen to lie parallel side by side or are twisted in strands like those of a rope —sometimes they have a plaited arrangement. These bundles twist about and cross in all directions, and eventually disappear at the periphery of the colony. The colony itself is not circumscribed in its appearance, but is more or less irregularly fringed and ragged, or scalloped. To the naked eye they look very much like minute pellicles of raw cotton which had been pressed into the surface of the agar-agar. At the extreme periphery of the colonies it is sometimes possible to trace single bundles of these threads for long distances across the surface of the agar-agar.

As the colonies continue to grow, they become more and more dense; they become opaque in color, and granular and rough on the surface. When touched with a sterilized needle, one experiences a sensation that suggests, somewhat, the matted structure of these colonies. The bit that may thus be taken from a colony is always more or less ragged.

GELATIN.—The colonies on gelatin at the earliest stages also present the same wavy appearance; but this characteristic soon becomes in part destroyed by the liquefaction of the gelatin which is produced by the growing organisms. This allows them to sink to the bottom of the fluid, where they lie as an irregular mass. Through the fluid portion of the gelatin may be seen small clumps of growing bacilli, which look very much like bits of cotton-wool.

BOUILLON.—In bouillon the growth is characterized by the formation of flaky masses, which also have very much the appearance of bits of cotton. Microscopic examination of one of these flakes shows the twisted and plaited arrangement of the long threads.

POTATO.—It develops rapidly as a dry, granular, whitish mass, which is more or less limited to the point of inoculation. On potato, at the temperature of the incubator, its spore-formation may easily be observed.

STAB AND SLANT CULTURES.—Stab and slant cultures on agar-agar present in general the appearances given for the colonies, except that the growth is much more extensive. The growth is always more pronounced on the surface than down the track of the needle.

On gelatin it causes liquefaction, which begins on the surface at the point inoculated, and spreads outward and downward.

It grows best with access to oxygen, and very poorly when the supply of oxygen is interfered with.

Under favorable conditions of oxygen, nutrition, and temperature its growth is rapid.

Under 12° C. and above 45° C. no growth occurs. The temperature of the body is most favorable to its development. The spores of the anthrax bacillus are very resistant to heat, though the degree of resistance is seen to vary with spores of different origin. Esmarch found that anthrax spores from one source would readily be killed by an exposure of one minute to the temperature of steam, whereas those from other sources resisted this temperature for longer times, reaching in some cases as long as twelve minutes.

STAINING.—The anthrax bacilli stain readily with the ordinary aniline dyes. In tissues their presence may also be demonstrated by the ordinary aniline staining fluids, or by Gram's method. They may also be stained in tissues with a strong watery solution of dahlia, after which the tissue is decolorized in 2 per cent. soda solution, washed in water, dehydrated in alcohol, cleared up in xylol, and mounted in balsam. This leaves the bacilli stained, while the tissues are decolorized; or the tissues may be stained a contrast color—eosin, for example—after the dehydration in alcohol, and before the clearing up in xylol. In this case they must be washed out again in alcohol before using the xylol. In the preparation treated in this way, the rod-shaped organisms will be of a purple color, and will be seen in the capillaries of the tissues, while the tissues themselves will be of a pale-rose color.

INOCULATION INTO ANIMALS.—Introduce into the subcutaneous tissues of the abdominal wall of a guinea-pig or rabbit, a portion of a pure culture of the bacillus anthracis. In about forty-eight hours the animal will be found dead. Immediately at the point of inoculation but little or no reaction will be noticed, but beyond this, extending for a long distance over the abdomen and thorax, the tissues will be markedly œdematous. Here and there, scattered through this œdematous tissue, small ecchymoses will be seen. The underlying muscles are pale in color. Inspection of the internal viscera reveals no very marked macroscopic changes except in the spleen. This is enlarged, dark in color, soft and brittle. The liver may present the appearance of cloudy swelling; the lungs may be pale or pale-red in color; the heart is usually filled with blood. There are no other changes to be seen by the naked eye. Prepare cover-slip preparations from the blood and other viscera. They will all be found to contain the short rods in large numbers. Nowhere can spore-formation be detected. Upon microscopic examination of sections of the organs which have been hardened in alcohol, the capillaries are seen to be filled with the bacilli; in some places closely packed together in large numbers, at other points fewer in number. Usually they are present in largest numbers in those tissues having the greatest capillary distribution and at those points at which the circulation is slowest. They are moderately evenly distributed through the spleen. The glomeruli of the kidneys and the capillaries of the lungs are frequently quite packed with them. The capillaries of the liver contain them in large numbers. Hemorrhages, probably due to rupture of capillaries by the mechanical pressure of the bacilli which are developing in them, not uncommonly occur. When this occurs in the mucous membranes of the alimentary tract, the blood may escape through the mouth or anus; when in the kidneys, through the uriniferous tubules.

Cultures from the different organs or from the œdematous fluid about the point of inoculation, result in growth of the bacillus anthracis.

The amphibia, dogs, and the majority of birds are not susceptible to this disease. Rats are difficult to infect. Rabbits, guinea-pigs, white mice, gray house-mice, sheep, and cattle are susceptible. Infection may occur either through the circulation, through the air-passages, through the alimentary tract, or, as we have just seen, through the subcutaneous tissues.

EXPERIMENTS.

Prepare three cultures of anthrax bacilli—one upon gelatin, one upon agar-agar, and one upon potato. Allow the gelatin culture to remain at the ordinary temperature of the room, place the agar culture in the incubator, and the potato culture at a temperature not above 18° to 20° C. Prepare cover-slips from each from day to day. What differences are observed?

Prepare two potato cultures of the anthrax bacillus. Place one in the incubator and retain the other at a temperature of from 18° to 20° C. Examine them each day. Do they develop in the same way?

From a fresh culture of anthrax bacilli, in which spore-formation is not yet begun, prepare a hanging-drop preparation; also a cover-slip preparation in the usual way and stain it with a strong gentian-violet solution, and another cover-slip preparation which will be drawn through the flame twelve to fifteen times, stained with aniline gentian-violet, washed off in iodine solution, and then in water. Examine these microscopically. Do they all present the same appearance? To what are the differences due?

Do the anthrax threads, as seen in a fresh, growing hanging drop, present the same morphological appearance as when dried and stained upon a cover-slip? How do they differ?

Liquefy a tube of agar-agar, and when it is at the temperature of 40° to 43° C., add a very minute quantity of an anthrax culture which is far advanced in the spore stage. Mix it thoroughly with the liquid agar-agar and from this prepare several hanging drops under strict antiseptic precautions, using the fluid agar-agar for the drops instead of bouillon or salt solution. Select from among these preparations that one in which the smallest number of spores are present. Under the microscope observe the development of this spore into a mature cell. Describe carefully the steps.

Prepare a 1 : 1000 solution of carbolic acid in bouillon. Inoculate this with virulent anthrax spores. If no development occurs after two or three days at the temperature of the thermostat, prepare a solution of 1 : 1200, and continue until the point is reached at which the amount of carbolic acid present just admits of the development of the spores. When the proper dilution is reached prepare a dozen of such tubes and inoculate one of them with virulent anthrax spores. As soon as development is well advanced transfer a loopful from this tube into a second of the carbolic acid tubes; when this has developed, then from this into a third, etc. After five or six generations which have been treated in this way, study the spore-production of the organisms in that tube. If it is normal, continue to inoculate from one carbolic acid tube into another, and see if it is possible by this means to influence in any way the production of spores by the organism with which you are working. What is the effect, if any?

Prepare two bouillon cultures, each from *one drop* of blood of an animal dead of anthrax. Allow one of them to grow for from fourteen to eighteen hours in the incubator; the other allow to grow at the same temperature for three or four days. Remove the first after the time mentioned and subject it to a temperature of 80° C. for thirty minutes. At the end of this time prepare four plates from it. Make each plate with one drop from the heated bouillon culture. At the end of three or four days treat the second tube in identically the same way. How do the number of colonies which developed from the two different cultures compare? Was there any difference in the time required for their development on the plates?

From a potato culture of anthrax bacilli which has been in the incubator for three or four days, scrape away the growth and carefully break it up in 10 c.c. of sterilized normal salt solution. The more carefully it is broken up the more accurate will be the experiment. Place this in a bath of boiling water and at the end of one, three, five, seven, and ten minutes make a plate upon agar-agar with one ocsc of the contents of this tube. Are the results on the plates alike?

EXPERIMENTS.

Determine the exact time necessary to sterilize objects, such as silk or cotton threads, on which anthrax spores have been dried, by the steam method and by the hot-air method.

Prepare from the blood of an animal just dead of anthrax a bouillon culture. After this has been in the incubator for, from three to four hours, subject it to a temperature of 55° C. for ten minutes. At the end of this time make plates from it, and also inoculate a rabbit subcutaneously with it. What are the results? Are the colonies on the plates in every way characteristic?

Inoculate six Erlenmeyer flasks of sterile bouillon, each containing about 35 c c. of the medium, from either the blood of an animal just dead of anthrax or from a fresh virulent culture in which *no spores* are formed.

Place these flasks in the incubator at a temperature of 42.5° C. At the end of five, ten, fifteen, twenty, twenty-five, etc., days remove a flask. Label each flask as it is taken from the incubator with the exact number of days for which it had been at the temperature of 42.5° C. Study each flask carefully, both in its cultural peculiarities and its pathogenic properties, when employed on animals.

Are these cultures identical in all respects with those that have been kept at 37° C.?

If they differ, in what respect is the difference most conspicuous?

Should any of the animals survive the inoculations made from the different cultures in the foregoing experiment, note carefully which one it is, and after ten to twelve days repeat the inoculation, using the same culture; if it again survives, inoculate it with the culture preceding the one just used in the order of removal from the incubator; if it still survives, inoculate it with virulent anthrax. What is the result? How is the result to be explained? Do the cultures which were made from these flasks at the time of their removal from the incubators act in the same way toward animals as the organisms growing in the flasks? Is the action of each of these cultures the same for mice, guinea-pigs, and rabbits?

Prepare a 2 per cent. solution of sulphuric acid in distilled water; suspend in this a number of anthrax spores; at the end of three, six, and nine days at 35° C. inoculate both a guinea-pig and a rabbit. Prepare cultures from this suspension on the third, sixth, and ninth days; when the cultures have developed inoculate a rabbit and a guinea-pig from the culture made on the ninth day. Should the animal survive, inoculate it again after three or four days with a culture made on the sixth day. Do the results appear in any way peculiar?

CHAPTER XXIV.

Bacteriology of diphtheria—Behavior of the bacillus diphtheriæ in the tissues of susceptible animals.

FROM the gray-white deposit on the fauces of a diphtheritic patient prepare a series of cultures in the following way:

Have at hand five or six tubes of Löffler's blood-serum mixture. (See article on Media.)

Pass a stout platinum needle, which has been sterilized, into the membrane and twist it around once or twice or brush it gently over the surface of the membrane. Without touching it against anything else smear it carefully over the surface of one of the serum tubes; without sterilizing it pass it over the surface of the second, then the third, fourth, and fifth tube. Place these tubes in the incubator. Then prepare cover-slips from scrapings from the membrane on the fauces. If the case is true diphtheria the tubes will be ready for examination on the following day.

The reason that plates are not made in the regular way in this experiment is that the bacillus of diphtheria develops much more luxuriantly on the serum-mixture, from which plates cannot be made, than it does on the media from which they can be made. The method employed, however, insures a dilution in the number of organisms present, and this, in addition to the fact that the bacillus diphtheriæ grows much more quickly on the serum mixture than do other organisms, makes its isolation by this method a matter of but little difficulty.

After twenty-four hours in the incubator the tubes will present a characteristic appearance. Their surfaces will be marked here and there by more or less irregular patches of a dense white or cream-colored growth which is usually more dense at the centre than at its irregular periphery.

Except now and then when a few orange-colored colonies may be seen, these large irregular patches are the most conspicuous objects on the surface of the serum. Now and then almost nothing else can be made out on the tubes.

The cover-slips made from the membrane at the time the cultures were prepared will be found in many cases to present a great variety of organisms, but conspicuous among them will be noticed slightly curved bacilli of very irregular size and outline. In some cases they will be more or less clubbed at one or both ends; sometimes they appear spindle in shape, again as curved wedges; now and then they will be seen irregularly segmented. They are rarely or never regular in outline. If the preparation has been stained with Löffler's alkaline methylene-blue solution many of these irregular rods are seen to be marked by circumscribed points in their protoplasm which stain very intensely; they appear almost black. This irregularity in outline is the morphological characteristic of the bacillus diphtheriæ of Löffler. It must be remembered, however, that the diagnosis of diphtheria cannot be made from the examination of cover-slip preparations alone, for there are other organisms present in the mouth cavity, particularly in the mouth of those having decayed teeth, the morphology of which is so like that of the bacillus of diphtheria that they might easily be mistaken for that organism if subjected to microscopic examination alone.

The bacillus diphtheriæ of Löffler (its discoverer) can readily be identified by its cultural peculiarities in connection with its pathogenic activity when introduced into tissues of susceptible animals. In guinea-pigs and kittens the results of its growth are identical with those found in the bodies of human beings who have died of diphtheria.

When studied in pure culture, its morphological and cultural peculiarities are as follows:

In morphology it varies greatly in size and shape, averaging 2.5 to 3 μ in length and 0.5 to 0.8 μ in thickness. Its morphological characters are so peculiar as to render its detection on cover-slip preparations, and in sections from diphtheritic membranes, in most cases an easy matter. Sometimes appearing as a regular straight or slightly bent rod, with rounded ends, it is especially characteristic to find irregular, bizarre forms, such as rods with one or both ends swollen, and very frequently rods broken at irregular intervals into short, sharply marked segments, either round, oval, or with straight sides. Some forms stain uniformly, others in various irregular ways, the most common being the appearance of deeply stained granules in a lightly stained bacillus.

GROWTH ON SERUM-MIXTURE.—The medium upon which it grows most rapidly and luxuriantly, and which is best adapted for determining its presence in diphtheritic exudations is, as has been stated, the blood-serum mixture of Löffler. (See chapter on Media.) On the blood-serum mixture the colonies of the bacillus diphtheriæ grow so much more rapidly than other organisms usually present in the secretious and exudations in the throat that at the end of twenty-four hours they are often the only colonies that attract attention, and if others of similar size are present, they are generally of quite a different aspect Its colonies are large, round, elevated, grayish-white, with a centre more opaque than the slightly irregular periphery. The surface of the colony is at first moist, but after a day or two rather dry in appearance.

A blood-serum tube studded over with coalescent or scattered colonies of this organism is so characteristic in appearance that one can anticipate with tolerable certainty the results of microscopic examination.

GLYCERIN AGAR-AGAR.—Upon nutrient glycerin-agar-agar the colonies likewise present an appearance which may readily be recognized. They are in every way more delicate in their structure than when on the serum mixture. They appear at first, when on the surface, as very flat, almost transparent, dry, non-glistening, round, points which are not elevated above the surface upon which they are growing. When slightly magnified they are seen to be granular, and present an irregular central marking which is more dense and darker by transmitted light than the thin, delicate zone which surrounds it. The periphery of the colony is marked by an irregularly notched appearance. These colonies are always quite dry in appearance. When deep down in the agar-agar they are coarsely granular. They rarely exceed 3 mm. in diameter.

GELATIN.—On gelatin the colonies develop much more slowly than on the other media which can be retained at a higher temperature. They rarely present their characteristic appearances on gelatin in less than seventy-two hours.

They then appear as flat, dry, translucent points, usually round in outline.

When magnified slightly, the centre is seen to be more dense than the surrounding zone or zones, for they are sometimes marked by a concentric arrangement of zones. The periphery is irregularly notched. Like the colonies seen on agar-agar, they are granular, but are much more granular when seen in the depths of the gelatin than when on its surface. On gelatin the colonies rarely become very large; usually they do not reach a diameter of over 1.5 mm.

BOUILLON.—In bouillon it usually grows in fine clumps, which fall to the bottom of the tube, or become deposited on its sides without causing a diffuse clouding of the bouillon. There are sometimes exceptions to this naked-eye appearance. The bouillon may appear diffusely clouded, but if one inspects it very closely, particularly if one examines it microscopically in the form of a hanging drop, the arrangement in clumps will still be seen, but they are so small as not to have been detected by the unaided eye.

In bouillon which is kept at a temperature of 35°-37° C. for a long time, a soft, whitish membrane often forms over a part of the surface.

Changes in Reactions of the Bouillon.—The reaction of the bouillon becomes at first acid, and, subsequently, again alkaline, changes which can be well observed in cultivations in bouillon to which a little rosolic acid has been added.

POTATO.—On potato at a temperature of 35°-37° C. its growth after several days is entirely invisible; only a thin, dry glaze can be noticed at the point at which the potato was inoculated. Microscopic examination of the potato after twenty-four hours at 35°–37° C. shows a decided increase in the number of individual organisms planted.

STAB AND SLANT CULTURES.—In stab and slant cultures on both gelatin and glycerin agar-agar, the surface growth is seen to predominate over that along the track of the needle in the depths of the media.

Isolated colonies on the surface of either of the media in this method of cultivation present the same characteristics that have been given for the colonies.

The growth in simple stab cultures does not extend laterally very far beyond the point at which the needle entered the medium.

It is a non-motile organism.

It does not form spores.

It is killed in ten minutes by a temperature of 58° C.

It grows at temperatures ranging from 22° C. to 37° C., but most luxuriantly at the latter temperature.

Its growth in the presence of oxygen is more active than when the gas is excluded.

STAINING.—In cover-slip preparations made either from the fauces of a diphtheritic patient, or from a pure culture of the organism, it is seen to stain readily with the ordinary aniline dyes. It stains also by the method of Gram, but the best results are those obtained by the use of Löffler's alkaline methylene-blue solution; this brings out the dark points in the protoplasmic body of the bacilli and aids thus in their identification.

For the purpose of demonstrating the Löffler bacilli in sections of diphtheritic membrane, both the Gram method and the fibrin method of Weigert give excellent results.

PATHOGENIC PROPERTIES.—When inoculated subcutaneously into the bodies of susceptible animals the result is not the production of a septicæmia as is seen to follow the introduction into animals of certain other organisms with which we shall have to deal. The bacillus of diphtheria remains localized at the point of inoculation, never spreading further than the nearest lymphatic glands. It develops at the point in the tissues at which it is deposited, and during its development gives rise to changes in the tissues which result entirely from the absorption into the circulation of poisonous albumins produced by the bacilli in the course of their development.

If a very minute portion of either a solid or fluid pure culture of this organism is introduced into the subcutaneous tissues of a guinea-pig or kitten, death of the animal is seen to ensue in from twenty-four hours to five days. The usual changes are an extensive local œdema with more or less hyperæmia and ecchymosis at the site of inoculation; frequently swollen and reddened lymphatic glands; increased serous fluid in the peritoneum, pleura, and pericardium; enlarged and hemorrhagic supra-renal capsules; occasionally slightly swollen spleen; sometimes fatty degeneration in the liver, kidney, and myocardium. The bacilli are always to be found at the seat of inoculation, most abundant in the grayish-white fibrino-purulent exudate present at the point of inoculation, and becoming fewer at a distance from this, so that the more remote parts of the œdematous fluid do not contain any bacilli. The bacilli are found not only free, but contained in large number in leucocytes, some of which have fragmented nuclei or have lost their nuclei. The bacilli within the leucocytes as well as some outside frequently stain very faintly and irregularly, and may appear disintegrated and dead.

In all cases culture-tubes inoculated with the blood, spleen, liver, kidneys, supra-renal capsules, distant lymphatic glands, and serous transudates yield negative growths. Negative results are also always obtained when these organs are examined microscopically for the bacilli.

Microscopic examinations of the tissues about the seat of inoculation, as well as of the liver, spleen, kidneys, lymphatic glands, and elsewhere, show a condition of extensive cell-death which is characterized by an extreme degree of fragmentation of the nuclei of the cells of these parts. These peculiar alterations, as Oertel has shown, in their distribution are characteristic of human diphtheria, and the demonstration of similar changes in animals inoculated with this organism is no small additional proof that diphtheria is caused by it.

An affection may be produced by the inoculation of certain animals in all respects identical with the disease diphtheria as it exists in man. If one opens the trachea of a kitten and rubs upon the mucous membrane a small portion of a pure culture of this organism, the death of the animal will ensue in from two to four days. At autopsy the wound will be found covered with a grayish, adherent, necrotic, distinctly diphtheritic layer. Around the wound the subcutaneous tissues will be œdematous. The lymphatic glands at the angle of the jaws will be swollen and reddened. The mucous membrane of the trachea at the point upon which the bacilli were deposited will be covered with a tolerably firm, grayish-white, loosely attached pseudo-membrane in all respects identical with the croupous membrane observed in the same situation in cases of human diphtheria. In the pseudo-membrane and in the œdematous fluid about the skin-wound, bacilli diphtheriæ may be found both in cover-slips and in cultures.

From what we have seen—the localization of the bacilli at the point of inoculation, their absence from the internal organs, and the changes brought about in the cellular elements of the internal organs—there is but one interpretation for this process, and that is the production of a soluble poison by the bacteria growing at the seat of inoculation, which gains access to the circulation and produces the changes that we observe in the tissues of the internal viscera.

This poison has been isolated from cultures of the bacillus of diphtheria by Brieger and Fränkel. It is found to belong, not to the crystallizable ptomaines, but to the toxic albumins. By the introduction of this toxalbumin, as it is called, into the tissues of guinea-pigs and rabbits the same pathological alterations may be produced that we have seen to follow the result of inoculation with the bacilli themselves, except, perhaps, the production of false membrane.

Prepare cover-slip preparations from the mouth cavity of healthy individuals and from those having decayed teeth. Do they correspond in any way with those made from diphtheria? Do the same with different forms of sore-throat. Do the peculiarities of any of the organisms suggest those of the bacillus of diphtheria? Wherein is the difference?

In cultures and cover-slips made from both diphtheria

and innocent sore-throats are there any organisms which are almost constantly present? Which are they, and what are their characteristics?

In the anginas of scarlet fever which are the predominating organisms?

In their cultural and morphological peculiarities, do these organisms simulate any of the different species with which you have been working?

CHAPTER XXV.

Experiments illustrating precautions to be taken in the study of disinfectants and antiseptics—Skin disinfection.

INTO each of three tubes containing 10 c.c.—one of normal salt solution, another of bouillon, a third of fluid blood-serum—add as much of a culture of the staphylococcus pyogenes aureus as can be held upon the looped platinum needle. Mix this thoroughly, so that no clumps exist, and then add exactly 10 c.c. of 1:500 solution of corrosive sublimate. Mix it thoroughly, and at the end of three minutes transfer a drop from each tube into a tube of liquefied agar-agar, and pour this into a Petri dish. Label each dish carefully and place them in the incubator. Are the results the same in all the plates? How are the differences to be explained?

Into each of two tubes containing 10 c.c.—the one of normal salt solution, the other of bouillon—add as much of a spore-containing culture of anthrax bacilli as can be held upon the loop of the platinum wire. Mix this thoroughly so that no clumps exist and then add exactly 10 c.c. of a 1:500 solution of corrosive sublimate. Mix thoroughly and at the end of five minutes transfer a drop from each tube into a tube of liquefied agar-agar. Pour this immediately into a Petri dish. Label each dish carefully and place them in the incubator. Note the results at the end of twenty-four, forty-eight, and seventy-two hours. How do you explain them?

Make identically the same experiment with a spore-containing culture of anthrax, except that the drop from the mixture will be transferred to 10 c.c. of a mixture of equal parts of ammonium sulphide and sterilized distilled water. After remaining in this for about half a minute, a drop will be transferred to a tube of liquefied agar-agar, poured into Petri dishes, labelled, and placed in the incubator. Note the results. How are they explained?

Prepare a 1 : 1000 solution of corrosive sublimate. To each of twelve bouillon tubes containing exactly 10 c.c. add: one drop to the first one, two drops to the second, and so on until the last tube has had twelve drops added to it. Mix thoroughly and then inoculate each with one wire loopful of a bouillon culture of staphylococcus pyogenes aureus. Place them all in the incubator after carefully labelling them. Note the order in which growth appears.

Do the same with anthrax spores, with spores of bacillus subtilis, with the typhoid bacillus, and see how the results compare. From these experiments what will be the strength of corrosive sublimate necessary to act as an antiseptic under these conditions for the organisms employed?

Make a similar series of experiments, using a five per cent. solution of carbolic acid.

Determine the antiseptic point in bouillon of the common disinfectants for the organisms with which you are working.

Determine the time necessary for the destruction of the organisms with which you are working, by corrosive sublimate in 1 : 1000 solution, under different conditions—with and without the presence of albuminous bodies other than the bacteria and under varying conditions of temperature.

In making these experiments be careful to guard against the introduction of enough sublimate into the agar-agar from which the Petri plate is to be made to inhibit the growth of the organisms which may not have been destroyed by the sublimate. This may be done by transferring two drops from the mixture of sublimate and organisms into not less than 10 c.c. of sterilized salt solution in which they may be thoroughly shaken for from one to two minutes, or into the solution of ammonium sulphide of the strength given.

To 10 c.c. of a bouillon culture of staphylococcus pyogenes aureus, or anthrax spores, add 10 c.c. of corrosive sublimate in 1 : 500 solution, and allow it to remain in contact with the organisms for *only one-half* the time necessary to destroy them (use an organism for which this has been determined under these conditions). Then transfer a drop of the mixture to each of three liquefied agar-agar tubes and pour them into Petri dishes. Place them in the incubator and observe them for twenty-four, forty-eight, and seventy-two hours. No growth occurs. How is this to be accounted for?

At the end of seventy-two hours inoculate all of these plates with a culture of the same organism which has not been exposed to sublimate, by taking up bits of the culture on the needle and drawing it across the plates. A growth now results. We have here an experiment in which organisms which have been exposed to sublimate for a much shorter time than is necessary to destroy them, when transferred directly to a culture medium do not grow, and yet, when the same organism which has not been exposed to sublimate is planted upon the same medium it does grow. How is this to be accounted for?

SKIN-DISINFECTION.—With a sterilized knife scrape from the skin of the hands, at the root of the nails and under the nails, small particles of epidermis. Prepare plates from them. Note the results.

Wash the hands carefully for ten minutes in hot water and scrub them during this time with soap and a sterilized brush. Rinse them in hot water. Again prepare plates from scrapings of the skin on the fingers, at the root of the nails, and under the nails. Note the results.

Again wash as before in hot water with soap and brush, rinse in hot water, then soak the hands for five minutes in 1:1000 corrosive sublimate solution, and, as before, prepare plates from scrapings from the same localities. Note the results.

Repeat this latter procedure in exactly the same way, but before taking the scrapings let someone pour ammonium sulphide over the points from which the scrapings are to be made. After it has been on the hands about three minutes again scrape and note the results upon plates made from the scrapings.

Wash as before in hot water and soap, rinse in clean hot water, immerse for a minute or two in alcohol, after this in 1:1000 sublimate solution, and finally in ammonium sulphide, and then prepare plates from scrapings from the points mentioned.

In what way do the results of these experiments differ the one from the other?

To what are these differences due?

What have these experiments taught?

In making the above experiments it must be remembered that the strictest care is necessary in order to prevent the access of germs from without into our media. The hand upon which the experiment is being performed must be held away from the body and must not touch any object not concerned in the experiment. The scraping should be done with the point of a knife which has been sterilized in the flame and allowed to cool down. The scrapings may be transferred directly from the knife-point to the gelatin by means of a sterilized platinum wire loop.

The brush used should be thoroughly cleansed and always kept in 1 : 1000 solution of corrosive sublimate. It should be washed in hot water before using.

INDEX.

ABSCESSES, miliary, 221
 microscopic appearances of, 222, 223
Aërobic organisms, 28
Agar-agar, 57, 65
 clarification of, 65
 filtration of, 66
 peculiarities of, 57, 58
Air, bacteriological analysis of, 186
 Petri's method for, 187
 Sedgwick's method for, 187–191
Anaërobic organisms, 27, 28
 methods of cultivation, 116–119
 method of Buchner, 117
 Esmarch, 119
 Fränkel, 118
 Hesse, 117
 Kitasato and Weil, 119
 Koch, 117
 Liborius, 119
Aniline dyes as aids in differentiation, 115
Animals, inoculation of, 151–158
 intra-venous, 154–158
 instruments for, 156–158
 subcutaneous, 151
 post-mortem examination of, 159–163
 cultures from tissues, 161
 disinfection of implements, 163
 disposal of remains, 163
 external inspection, 159
 incision through skin, 159
 opening the cavities, 160
 position of the animal, 159

Anthrax, 232
 bacillus of, 232–238
 cultivation of, 234–236
 experiments with, 238–242
 inoculation with, 236–238
 staining of, 236
Antiseptics, 53
 experiments upon, 254
Apparatus for air analysis, Petri's, 187
 Sedgwick's 188
 for counting colonies, Esmarch's, 184
 Wolffhügel's, 182
Autoclav or digestor, 46

BACILLI, 29–32
 Bacillus subtilis, 173
 of tuberculosis, 211
Bacteria, capsule surrounding, 133
 classification of, 29
 constant characteristics of, 104
 definition of, 22
 flagellæ upon, 136
 isolation of, on solid media, 54
 Koch's observation, 54–57
 microscopic examination of, 105
 morphology of, 29
 constancy of, 31
 motility of, 36
 multiplication of, 32, 33
 nutrition of, 25–27

INDEX.

Bacteria, reactions produced by, 114
  relation to oxygen, 27, 28
  to staining reagents, 115
  to temperature, 28
  rôle in nature, 23-25
  systematic study of, 104-121
    scheme for, 164, 165
Bacterium coli commune, 230, 231
Benches, glass, for holding plates, 85
Blood-serum, 69
  Löffler's mixture, 75, 76
  preparation of, 69
  preservation of, 73, 74
  solidification of, 71-73
  sterilization of, 71
Bonnet, 20
Bottles for staining solutions, 128
Bouillon, 57-59
  neutralization of, 60, 61
Box, iron, in which to sterilize plates, 84
Brownian motion, 110
Bulb for water samples, 179
Burner, Koch's safety, 93, 94
  rose or crown, 47

CHLOROPHYLL, definition of, 22
Cohn, 20
Colonies, characteristic appearance of, 168, 169
  study of, 99-101
Cooling-stage, 84
Cover-slips, cleaning of, 123
  impression, 126
  microscopic examination of, 107
  preparation of, 123-127
  steps in making, 124
Culture-dish for plates, 85
Cultures, gelatin, 113
  hanging-drop, 109
  potato, 113
    in tube, 69
  pure, 101
  stab and smear, 101-103
    method of making, 101, 102

DECOLORIZING solutions, 139
  Decomposition, 22, 23
Diphtheria, 243
  bacillus of, 245-252
  cultivation of, 245-248
  pathogenic properties of, 249-252
  preparation of cultures from, 243-245
  staining of, 248
Diplococci, 30
Diplococcus of pneumonia, 194
Disinfectants, experiments upon, 253-257
Disinfection, 49-53
  agents employed for, 52, 53
  in the laboratory, 52
  inorganic salts for, 49-51
  methods of, 52

ERYSIPELAS, 224
  Esmarch's roll tubes, 87
  modification of Esmarch's method, 88
  advantages of this process, 89
  roll tubes of agar-agar, 89
  tube being rolled on ice, 88
Experiments, 167
  exposure and contact, 169, 170

FACULTATIVE aërobic and anaërobic organisms, 28
Fermentation, 22, 23, 116
Filters, preparation of, 64
Flagellæ, Löffler's method of staining, 136
Flasks, etc., cleaning of, 77
Funnel for filling Sedgwick's aërobioscope, 190
  for filling test-tubes, etc., 79

GELATIN, 57-62
  clarification of, 63
  filtration of, 63
  peculiarities of, 57, 58
Guarniari's agar-gelatin, 76

INDEX.

HANGING-DROP preparations, 108
Henle, 17
Hoffmann, 19
Hypodermatic needles, 156
    syringes, 158

INCUBATORS, 91–93
Indol, its production by bacteria, 120
    method for detecting its presence, 120, 121
Introduction, 13

LEEUWENHOEK'S discoveries, 13–15
Lens for counting colonies, 183
Levelling tripod, 84
Löffler's blood-serum mixture, 75, 76

MEDIA, 59–76
  agar-agar, 65–67
    clarification of, 65, 66
    filtration of, 66
    solution of, 65, 66
  blood-serum, 69–74
    precautions in obtaining, 69, 70
    preservation of, 73, 74
    solidifying, 71–73
    sterilization of, 71
  bouillon, 59
    neutralization of, 59–61
  gelatin, 62–65
    clarification of, 63, 64
    filtration of, 63
    neutralization of, 62
  meat infusion, 76
  potatoes, 67–69
    for test-tube cultures, 68
  special, 74–76
    agar-gelatin of Guarniari, 76
    blood-serum mixture of Löffler, 75
    Dunham's peptone solution, 75

Media, special: Dunham's peptone solution, with rosolic acid, 75
  milk, 74
    as a solid medium, 74, 75
    with litmus, 74
Micrococci, 29
Micrococcus of sputum septicæmia, 194–197
  tetragenus, 197
    animals susceptible to, 200
    description of, 198–200
    results of inoculation with, 197
Microscope, 105–107
  adjustment, coarse, 106
    fine, 106
  condenser, sub-stage, 106
  immersion system, oil, 106
    steps in using, 107
  objective, 105
  ocular, 105
  reflector, 106
  stage, 106
Microtome, 142
Mouse-holder, 152, 153

NEEDHAM, 18
Nitrites, 121

"OESE," platinum, 82
Oil-immersion system, steps in using, 107
Ozanam, 17

PARASITES, 22
Pasteur, 17–19
Pasteur and Chevreul, 19
Peptone solution, Dunham's, 75
  -rosolic-acid solution, 75
Petri's dish, 87
  modification of Koch's method, 86
Plates, technique of making, 81
Platinum needles, loops ("oese"), 81, 82
Plenciz, 16

Pneumococcus of Fränkel, 194
Potatoes, preparation of, 67
 for test-tube cultures, 68, 69
 sterilization of, 69
Practical application of bacteriological methods, 167
 materials for starting, 167
Pus organisms, 219-224

REGULATOR, gas-pressure, 97, 98
 thermo-, 94-97

SAPROPHYTES, definition of, 22
Sarciniæ, 30
Schröder and Dusch, 19
Schulz, 19
Schwann, 19
Section-cutting, 141
Septicæmia, definition of, 194
 sputum, 194
  organism concerned in, 195
  its different names, 194
  pathological alterations in, 194, 195
Skin-disinfection, experiments upon, 255-257
Soil, bacteriological study of, 191
Spallanzani, 18
Spirilli, 28-32
Spore-formation, 33-36
 study of, 110
  method for the, 111-113
Spores, staining of, 134
 Moeller's method, 135
Sputum, tubercular, 192
 microscopic examination of, 192
 results of inoculation with, 194-216
 septicæmia of micrococcus tetragenus, 197
 sputum septicæmia, 194
 tuberculosis, 201
Staining in general, 138
 methods of, 122-150

Staining solutions employed, 127
 bottles for, 128
 special solutions, 129-133
  acetic acid method, 133
  Gram's stain, 133
  Koch-Ehrlich, 129
  Löffler's blue, 129
  Ziehl's carbol fuchsin, 130
Staphylococci, 29
Staphylococcus pyogenes albus, 224
 aureus, 217
 citreus, 224
Sterilization, 37
 apparatus employed in, 43-47
 dry heat, 37
  its applications, 38
  experiments in, 171-175
  hot-air method, 174
  precautions, 171
  steam method, 171-174
  temperature in sterilizer, 171
 methods of, 39
  intermittent, at high temperature, 40, 41
  at low temperature, 41, 42
  under pressure, 42
 steam, 38
  its application, 39
Sterilizer, blood-serum, 72
 hot-air, 47
 steam, Arnold's, 45
  Koch's, 43
Streptococci, 29
Streptococcus pyogenes, 224
Suppuration, 217
 organisms concerned in acute, 219
 cultural peculiarities of, 217-219
 results of inoculation with, 219-223

TEST-TUBE cleaner, 77
Test-tubes, cleaning of, 77
 filling for Esmarch tubes, 80
  with media, 78, 79

Test-tubes, plugging with cotton, 78
  position after filling, 80
  sterilization after filling, 79
  sterilization of, 78
Tetrads, 30
Tissues, cultures from, 161
  hardening of, 141
  imbedding, 142
  staining of bacteria in, 140–143
    steps in the process, 145
    special methods of staining, 146
      dahlia method, 147
      dry method, 150
      Erhlich's method, 150
      Gram's method, 146
      Kühne's method, 148
      Weigert's method, 148
      Ziehl-Neelsen, 150
Tripod for levelling plates, 83
Tuberculosis, 201
  bacillus of, 211
  cultivation from the tissues, 212
  cultural peculiarities of, 213
  methods of staining, 131
    Nuttall's modification, 132
    dry method, 150
    Erhlich, 150
    Ziehl-Neelsen, 150
  microscopic appearance of, 214
  staining peculiarities of, 215
  cavity-formation, 206
  diffuse caseation, 205
  encapsulation of tubercular foci, 206

Tuberculosis, infection, modes of, 207
  primary, 206
  location of the bacilli in, 209
  manifestations of, 201–203
  miliary tubercles, 203
  susceptibility of animals to, 216
Tyndall, 20
Typhoid fever, 225
  bacillus of, 225–227
  in tissues, 227, 228
  results of inoculation with, 228–230

WATER, 176
  general observations upon bacteriological analysis of, 185
  qualitative bacteriological analysis of, 176
  precautions in obtaining samples for, 177
  preliminary steps in, 177
  quantitative bacteriological analysis of, 178
  counting the colonies in, 181
  apparatus for, 182, 183
  dilution of water for, 180, 181
  obtaining sample for, 179
  preliminary steps in, 180
  source of error in, 185
  relation to epidemics, 176
  typhoid organisms in, 230

ZOOGLŒA, 31

www.ingramcontent.com/pod-product-compliance
Lightning Source LLC
Chambersburg PA
CBHW021355230426
43666CB00006B/535